Asylum Histor

Buckinghamshire County
Pauper Lunatic Asylum–St John's

JOHN CRAMMER

Asylum History

Buckinghamshire County
Pauper Lunatic Asylum – St John's

GASKELL

Typeset by Dobbie Typesetting Limited, Tavistock, Devon
Printed in Great Britain

Contents

Figures

Tables

Preface

History is an account of human activities in the past, and there are two sorts of problems in presenting it. One is that it depends on written or printed records, and these can give only a partial, selected description of events. Even eyewitnesses are known to be unreliable, subjective in their perceptions, and any written account is inevitably subjective too, whether by design or unconscious bias. The whole truth in all its detail can never be known and history can only be written from what has been recorded.

The other problem is that the historian always has a purpose in writing a history (and readers likewise a purpose in reading it), and the author's purpose decides what he selects and emphasises in his account, the kind of order he imposes on the chaos of events. Medical history has frequently been written in terms of the lives and personalities of leaders, or of the advance of science and technology, or of the development of theoretical ideas; it is often imbued with the belief that things get progressively better as the ages go by, as in the current faith that the World Health Organization's "Health for All by 2000 A.D." is meaningful and attainable. This is to discount the effects of wars, famines, and religious beliefs of all kinds on human behaviour and to ignore the irrationality of 'group man'. The rise of sociology and Marxist belief has produced a different view of history, in which some influence is given to surges of mass emotion: the course of the past is seen as the struggles for power of different groups within the community.

Until about 30 years ago the history of psychiatry was left to medical men with a fondness for anecdote, a reverence for pioneers, and a belief in 'progress'. The medical reader's professional pride was warmed thereby – there was satisfaction in being the heir to such traditions. But then, led by the French philosopher Michel Foucault, a posse of non-medical sociologists and social historians rode onto the field. They declared that the doctors were simply a power-hungry professional clique which aimed to build up its social status and personal wealth by claiming exclusive domain over the mad, to the advantage of the establishment in maintaining a conservative social order. Doctors asserted that mad people were ill – mentally – and therefore should be treated on medical lines. The sociologists declared that psychiatry was a 'non-subject', and that the mad were simply social deviants, rebels against social conformity, antibourgeois, martyrs in the fight against capitalist oppression. The implication was that in a new, fairer society, madness would simply disappear as a kind of human behaviour requiring attention. Andrew Scull's *Museums of Madness* (1979; issued in paperback by Penguin in 1982) has been a widely published expression of this view of asylum history. The three volumes of *The Anatomy of Madness* (1985–88) edited by Bynum and Porter of the Wellcome Institute for the History of Medicine, with Shepherd, offer more scholarly presentations of antipsychiatric views.

There are two basic troubles with this sociological view. One is its inhumanity, if it is to be taken seriously. It advises us to distrust doctors, refuse drugs, and avoid hospitals, but offers nothing in their place. Those who are suffering, and their relatives who are suffering, must simply wait for the triumph of the new social order, and meanwhile go on suffering or die. This outlook is possible for the inhabitant of libraries and academic seminars who knows nothing of the realities of the clinic. People in fact flock to doctors and hospitals for help, and some at least seem satisfied thereby, whatever their drawbacks or errors. Is it not cruel to tell new sufferers to avoid what might help them?

More importantly, the ideas of Foucault and Scull, however intellectually original and productive of good PhD theses, simply do not fit the facts, in Britain at least. It has not been true for 50 years that patients in mental hospitals are mostly shut up against their will ('committed', 'certified', etc.). It is not true that there are no effective treatments, it is not true that no mental disturbances have a medical pathology and that no progress has been made in a hundred years of psychiatry. Nor is it true that English asylums were created as a form of oppression by the state. Nor till recently did doctors have much say in what went on in them; they were the servants of magistrates or county councillors. What happened in Buckinghamshire exemplifies the realities.

The view taken here of asylum history is that it is a resultant of the changing complexities of mental illness, the changes in technology brought to bear on it at different times, and the changing ways in which this area of life has been governed. What large groups of the population feel and believe at different times decide which individuals are to be specially handled. The technology – the buildings, the specialist staffs, the medical and therapeutic manoeuvres – determines the handling. Who gives the orders, and what orders they give to the staff, and how the staff interact among themselves in obeying, decide the outcomes. The history of an asylum is the history of the organisation and management, of who had the power and whether they used it with understanding, as well as the history of the conceptions of madness and the history of public attitudes to it. Viewed in this way the history is not propaganda for a new society, or a stick with which to beat the doctors, but a continuing display of human attitudes from which we learn more about the nature of man. By showing us the mistakes of the past it may also offer suggestions for the present, as with the history of any enterprise.

The plan of this book therefore is to set the social scene in the first two chapters, then to describe how an asylum was built, and to follow its running and management up to 1934, which was a turning point. Two chapters then discuss how the inmates were treated and by whom, and a further chapter analyses the good and bad results. The narrative then resumes with the development of a mental health service from the mental hospital (1935–48) and the expansion and upgrading of services under the National Health Service. The final chapter summarises 140 years of change, successes and failures, and the next steps in evolution.

Dr Julian Candy first suggested to me the writing of this history as St John's was about to close after 138 years. He allowed me to see all the annual reports, case books and journals of records kept since 1853. This was supplemented by committee minutes and other papers kept in the Bucks County Record Office in Aylesbury or in the library of the Oxford Regional Health Authority, where Mrs Enid Leonard was particularly helpful. My sister Mrs Sylvia Bradford assisted by interviewing a number of older, retired nurses, and I had the benefit of conversations with Dr S. L. Last and Dr D. C. Watt. Mr K. Nieland and the Oxford Regional Health Authority provided photographs. I am very grateful to them all, to Mrs Susan Floate (Librarian at the Royal College of Psychiatrists), and to other unnamed helpers, for information and useful suggestions. I remain fully responsible for the point of view and selection of material, and any errors there may be. I wanted to present a little-known piece of social history in readable form.

JC
Oxford, 1990

I. Social background

1 The nature of madness

The Buckinghamshire County Pauper Lunatic Asylum opened for the reception of patients on 17 January 1853. Over the next 130 years its government and its name was changed several times and the work it was expected to do changed also. It dropped the word 'pauper' in 1893, 'lunatic' in 1915, became 'County Mental Hospital' in 1919, and from the time it became part of the National Health Service in 1948 was called St John's Hospital, Stone.

Why was it built, what was it for, how well did it do its job? How did that job change? In some ways it resembled a boarding school, a big hotel, a monastery, a prison. That is, it was a group of people working together in a special building according to certain rules to provide a service to the community. How it was governed and financed, and how harmony was brought to the conflicting desires of the individuals who worked for it, are a part of social and political history, of English democracy, and easy to understand. But the particular service it rendered at different times is much harder to grasp. Because few people experienced it at first hand, the words used in talking about it remain foggy and unconnected with reality, and as horror, fear, and political passions frequently came in the door, sense and knowledge flew out the window.

Words

The words 'pauper', 'lunatic' and 'asylum' in the institution's original name are today open to great misunderstanding. For us, 'pauper' carries a flavour of extreme poverty and even of some moral disapproval – a person who is feckless, a social failure, perhaps a meths drinker sleeping rough under the arches – someone who might be tidied away in an institution of some kind. This was not the reality of 1853. A pauper asylum was one open without cost to patients or their families, and as such was provided for individuals by the community as a whole, something of a novelty in the early 19th century.

3

The troubles the asylum was there to help with might last a long time and people of modest means could not afford their true cost. The asylum could and did accept private fee-paying patients when it had room, but priority went to those who could not pay: farmers as well as labourers, clergy as well as clerks and small shopkeepers and navvies. When the Bucks County Council took over management after the Lunacy Act 1890 the word 'pauper' was dropped, and the place became simply a public asylum, which was what it always was.

'Asylum' is simply a sanctuary, a place of refuge or shelter offering protection from the harshness of life, but it now too often brings thoughts of life imprisonment under severe discipline and dirty, crowded conditions in some 'snake-pit', surrounded by terrifying companions, some wild and gibbering, and others wrongfully deprived of liberty for political or racial reasons. Well, of course such things have happened, and some have been the occasion of public inquiries. Whenever human beings are given power over others, whether in army, school, orphanage, or old people's home, that power is at times abused. Parliament has tried over and over again to enact laws and regulations to prevent such abuses, and 19th-century history is filled with such attempts, in particular to purify the private madhouses and similar institutions, which were sometimes gross offenders against humanity.

The public asylum was in its time one solution to these inhumanities and it set a high standard of care. Unfortunately the checks and safeguards so painfully created have later on occasion been thrown away by ignorant and forgetful people. The history of such institutions is therefore a fluctuating one, but there is little doubt that the good has outweighed the bad; the reader can judge from what follows as far as St John's Hospital, Stone, is concerned. Certainly, enormous efforts were made to avoid wrongful detention, and over a very long period about half those admitted to the asylum or hospital could expect to be home again within six months. On the other hand a proportion of the admissions was always elderly (over 65 years old) and in need of care, or younger chronically disabled people likewise needing care (perhaps because their parents had died), and such patients stayed the rest of their lives. It is important to realise what a mix of cases and problems the asylum took in. Simply to label them all as mad, without further inquiry, as some non-medical historians do (such as Andrew Scull (1979) in his *Museums of Madness*) is to fail to understand what the asylum was about. It was a refuge, a home from home, a place of cure, an adult school, a medical and surgical treatment centre, and more.

So what is a 'lunatic', a madman, a person of unsound mind? What are insanity, madness, mental illness? The madman was not a medical invention, but ordinary people's recognition that some human beings become *inexplicably* excited, or start talking to invisible persons and appear preoccupied by bizarre thoughts, or get fixed mistaken ideas beyond rational debate, and become incapable of work or activity, or even of caring for their own health and hygiene. Such people can be very difficult to live with. They may destroy part of the family home, or spend the family's money absurdly, or threaten to harm relations and neighbours, or attempt suicide. If ordinary life is to proceed they may have to be restrained in some way, at home, or by some private arrangement, or with the help of neighbours, or using a community resource such as a prison or workhouse. Such abnormal human beings are found all over the world, in all societies, in the USSR and in China, in India walled up in village houses, in Thailand chained to the corner post of the platform of a family home or in a strait-jacket loaned by the monks of some Buddhist temple. A high sheriff of Gloucestershire in England, Sir George Onesiphorus Paul, published in 1808 a famous letter about the state of the mad as he had seen them in England:

> "there is hardly a parish of any considerable size in which there may not be found some unfortunate human creature . . . chained in the cellar or garret of a workhouse, fastened to the leg of a table, tied to a post in an outhouse, or perhaps shut up in an uninhabited ruin." (Quoted from Jones, 1972, p. 56)

The asylum was a device to do better than that for the human unfortunates.

These obviously abnormal human beings are not so common, perhaps of the order of one in a thousand people only. In ordinary life we do not meet such people, but as soon as they begin to be collected together, as in an asylum, it becomes much easier to learn more about them, and this is what some of the medical men with the job of looking after them did. They perceived that madmen differed from one another in the nature of their abnormality. One might behave strangely because he was unutterably depressed, beyond all reason, while another felt obliged to do whatever spirit voices spoke to him to do, and a third might be extremely suspicious and aggressive to those around him. Descriptively one could look beyond the madness, the unreasonableness, to a more specific disturbance of normal feelings or logical thought or memory, and could observe how some individuals in the course of time got worse, others remained unchanging year after year, and yet others suddenly, surprisingly, recovered their normality. The mad came to be classified into people with different life patterns of mental illnesses, different futures and, eventually, different causes.

'Fever' is an old word for much physical illness. Today medically it is just one symptom in many different symptom groupings. We see fever as a part of many different bacterial infections (typhoid, pneumonia, meningitis, etc.), viral infections (measles, encephalitis, etc.) or protein allergies (e.g. hay fever) often particularly affecting one bodily organ. The concept of these distinctive diseases is useful in discovering the causes and the treatments for them. The same approach to madness yields mental illnesses, so called because their symptoms are mental, *not* because their causes (where known) are mental – in fact sometimes they are very obviously physical, for example, from smoking pot, or drinking alcohol, or a brain injury. A man is a single entity, a whole individual, not an immaterial soul clothed in a body like a jacket and trousers. Mind and body are but two aspects of the living person, and every illness has both a psychological (mental) and a physical side to it. Both may need treatment, depending on the balance of the case.

Observation of many cases has shown that psychological symptoms and different sorts of madness have regularities about their appearance and seem to follow rules. Thus detailed knowledge about them can be orderly, even logical, and this is the origin of the science of psychiatry. Because some mental disturbances recur with a monthly periodicity they were at one time ascribed to the influence of the recurrent full moon, and so the sufferers were 'lunatics' (*luna* = moon). Fuller knowledge has shown that monthly periodicity may not follow the moon's phases, nor for that matter the menstrual cycle: men, and women after the menopause, may have mental illness recurring every four weeks (but also every six weeks or three months, or some other period in different individuals).

People with mental illnesses have grown up as normal people and then something has gone wrong. But there are also people who have never from birth developed normally – the mentally defective, mentally retarded, mentally handicapped (different official labels at different times) – the most severely affected of whom are the idiots and imbeciles. Their ability to learn anything can be extremely slow, their understanding limited, their intelligence low, but they do not necessarily behave in a mad way. On the other hand a considerable number of them suffer from epilepsy and they are more liable than normal people to develop an adult type of mental illness later. In the right sheltered environment (e.g. a good family) they may behave very well, but they may be unusually intolerant of frustration, or easily upset, and may then act in a wild, aggressive, or mad way, but respond quickly to the right, friendly, understanding handling. Such episodes of wildness or tantrums may get them sent to hospital as mad, but their madness is quite different from the madness of the mentally ill and can often be abolished by social and simple psychological means. In 1853 they were admitted to the asylum along with the mentally ill, but later a separate service, with separate institutions, was developed for them.

In popular language the word 'mental' may be used to describe a person believed to be mad or someone thought to be seriously deficient in intelligence: the two states are often confused. A relative once said to me about a psychiatric in-patient with a psychotic illness, ''Of course I know he's not mental, doctor, it's only his nerves''. I am not sure what was meant: not 'mad' perhaps – that was true. But suffering from 'nerves' is a common lay phrase meaning there is something wrong in the head. Words such as 'lunatic', 'mad', 'unsound mind', 'nerves' no longer have precise meaning and are never used in medicine now.

The best way to understand what was meant by the word 'lunatic' in 1853 is to read descriptions of a few of the people brought into the County Pauper Lunatic Asylum in the first months after it opened. They came only because a magistrate or a clergyman of the parish recommended it, and a receiving officer or overseer of the poor had issued a certificate, and this was only likely where family or neighbours wanted it, or a person had been found wandering. Admission to the asylum was thus not a medical decision, but a lay judgement of 'madness', of a person's socially abnormal behaviour. The doctor could recommend that a person should be discharged home, but it was a committee of magistrates which formally allowed it.

Over the next 130 years the procedures and safeguards and the kinds of people who came to the asylum changed from time to time. It is necessary to keep in mind what sorts of people, what procedures, what purposes at this or that date, and not to assume that 'madness' or 'insanity' or 'mental home' always mean the same thing.

Sufferers

The following six brief case histories have been taken from a case book from the Buckingham County Pauper Lunatic Asylum from 1853. They are typical of the people then admitted. Similar cases would have been admitted to other asylums and the same kinds of case still turn up in modern psychiatry. There are of course many other kinds of case. Here are five men and one woman; the sex is irrelevant and accidental (these forms of madness affect both sexes) and are simply to give some idea of what a lunatic actually was in 1853.

Case 1

WE, a married man aged 57, was admitted to the asylum on Boxing Day 1853, because he had twice tried to kill himself. The first time, in August that year, he had cut his throat, but not effectively and it had been sewn up and had healed. Just before Christmas he got into the village pond to drown himself but was noticed and rescued, and now he had been sent for treatment. He told the doctor he had sinned past forgiveness, there was no hope for him, and he had no right to live. He refused all food, and he could not sleep at all at night.

> "It appears that this poor man has a wife and two children, one of whom is an idiot, that his wages have been only 8 shillings a week, and 9s when he worked on Sunday, a pittance so small (though the wages of the locality) that the parish is obliged to allow him three loaves a week to eke out a living till hay-time."

At first he had to be fed. Then he began to improve in spirits and put on weight, and began to work around the asylum. But he varied from day to day a good deal, sometimes active and friendly, sometimes much depressed and withdrawn, especially after visits from the clergyman of his parish, who reminded him he was needed at home. However, he lost his ideas of extreme sin and slept better, his recovery became solid and on 14 September, after about nine months, he was discharged to his home, with a gift of 20 shillings to pay for his first fortnight before he started work again.

Thus this man was sent to hospital to prevent him from killing himself, or through starvation falling seriously ill physically and perhaps dying. His mental illness consisted in his belief that he was a hopeless sinner and his inability to act in any way except suicidally; it disappeared in the asylum and did not recur when he went home. It was a very bad time of rural poverty (see Chapter 2), but other men did not behave in this way.

Case 2

JA, a single labourer aged 38, was admitted on 21 July, a ''thin anxious-looking man suffering from 'spectral illusions', the consequence of long-continued intemperance. He believes that snakes are crawling all over him and every now and then clutches hold of his body saying he has caught one''. He was said to have been a heavy drinker all his life, and at one time drank 147 pints of beer in 14 days.

In the asylum he was given three pints of beer daily and liquid nourishment, and in only two days he was much better. At four weeks he was noted to be working very well with the asylum bricklayer. He completely recovered and was discharged after six weeks.

This was a case of delirium tremens following excessive consumption of alcohol. The man was in a frightened, restless, uncomprehending state, in which he would not know where he was or who was with him; he needed calm and care until recovery.

Case 3

JE, a married man of 29 and a tailor by trade, was brought to the asylum on 1 October in a strait-jacket to control his violence: he had just attacked a neighbour with a poker. For about three weeks he had been very excited, running about from place to place, not doing anything or settling in one spot but getting into fights and talking incessantly. He was a tall, thin, haggard man who had twice been in prison for assault, and once sent to Bethlem Hospital in London for his mental disturbance. In the asylum he gradually calmed down, lost his irritability and aggressiveness, and by December was much improved. He went home fit in March 1854.

After about 18 months of normal life and work the attack of excitement came on again, and in a week he was back in the asylum: in on 9 November, out home again 27 March (1856). A further 18 months later he was quarrelsome, violent and restless once more, again unable to work: he was in the asylum from October 1857 to March 1858. He was well again until the autumn of 1859, but then he became very depressed, would not talk or show any activity, would not take food unless fed like a child, and hardly slept all night. Back in the asylum he quickly improved, and in three weeks became "industrious, free from excitement or depression, and coherent in conversation". He was home before Christmas 1859. About March 1861 he became depressed again, refusing to eat and wandering aimlessly, and was in the asylum till December. In 1864, 1865, 1867, 1869, and 1874 he was again admitted because of excitement and violence, lasting two to three months each time. After that there is no further record of him. Perhaps he committed suicide or died, or was imprisoned or sent to an asylum elsewhere. It seems unlikely that his recurrent illness would have ceased if he were alive.

The asylum prevented him from becoming agitated to the extent of showing people violence, or of wandering in a state of self-neglect and possibly starving. His mental illness consisted of overactivity without being able to concentrate on anything, or of excessive underactivity, and when restless in losing all control of his temper. Both over- and underactivity disappeared, given time, and he could then live a normal home and working life again.

Case 4

James E, aged 18, a baker, was a tall healthy-looking lad with a sad expression. He had been very attached to his mother, who had died when he was 15. For the year before admission in June 1853 he had become very apathetic. He stopped working, did nothing, and often refused to eat. He avoided any attempt at conversation. In the asylum he sat all day with his head on his arm, taking no notice of anything or anyone. He said his father must be somewhere in the asylum because he could hear his voice. He also complained that the canaries, which were in a cage in his ward, took his breath away, but did not explain this; he said he could not stand their noise. He kept his handkerchief over his mouth and spat frequently, as if trying to get rid of something.

Over the next four years he stayed in the asylum showing little change; occasionally he would eat and talk a little. His attacks of withdrawal became longer and more severe, however: "he suddenly becomes much lost and very stupid. Stands in one position all day long with a handkerchief over his mouth no entreaty getting him to utter a single word."

At the end of 1857, aged 22, he lost weight and began to cough and soon to spit blood. He died from pulmonary tuberculosis in April 1858.

The behavioural illness is obvious: inactivity such that he was unable to care for himself, as well as some strange ideas. The care he got was inadequate to prevent him catching and dying from tuberculosis, an asylum scourge for many years.

Case 5

ST, a very deaf widow washerwoman of 85, was transferred from the asylum at Devizes because she came from Newport Pagnell in Bucks and was therefore a Bucks responsibility. She had been a widow for 13 years and in an asylum for 7. She talked loudly to herself but because of her deafness could not hear a word said to her; this did not stop her from complaining that people talked to her all night and prevented her from sleeping. Sometimes she answered these voices. "At times she swore lustily at other patients because they called her a whore." She came to the Bucks asylum in February 1853, became feeble and bedridden in August, and died in April.

She sounds to have been cheerful and harmless enough, and if she had had a family to care for her she might have lived quite easily at home. But she had been left alone and without money and had initially been sent to end her days in the workhouse. There her restlessness at night and her swearing at the others by day had upset fellow members of her dormitory and made her a nuisance. The asylum was the place to tolerate her arguments with her hallucinatory voices.

Case 6

TS, a single man of 44, a sawyer, was transferred from prison on 26 April after being found guilty of murder. He had killed his grandfather in the next room at home. Since adolescence he had suffered from epilepsy and sometimes after a fit was slow to recover complete consciousness, and passed through a stage of automatic behaviour when he appeared fully awake but in fact had no knowledge or subsequent recollection of what actions he was taking. In the aftermath of an attack one night he had murdered his grandfather, without discoverable motive.

In the asylum he was described as frequently "lost", his mind a blank, and he was liable in this state to urinate or defaecate anywhere in the room. He was looked after, cleaned and fed, and prevented from hurting himself. He lived so for seven years, the fits gradually becoming more frequent: he was observed to have 250 in the last month of his life.

In major epilepsy there are episodic losses of consciousness, the sufferer falls to the ground, has a brief generalised stiffening of the muscles, followed by rhythmical jerking movements and then a short period of complete relaxation without breathing. Recovery to normal is usually swift and the sufferer continues with ordinary life. However, recovery in some is delayed and only partial, and a time of mental disturbance follows. Such people were quite likely to be brought to an asylum in Victorian times, when anti-epileptic drugs had not yet been discovered. Repeated uncontrolled fits damaged the brain and elderly epileptics often had to be cared for because they became demented, that is, lost their normal intelligence and power of memory. This man showed this late change.

These six people have in common an inability to get on with their everyday lives. They may be faced with one of the common misfortunes of life (poverty, deafness, loss of loved mother, and so on) but it is something inside them which has gone wrong, either temporarily or permanently, and which prevents them from coping. They make mistaken judgements, they misunderstand their experiences, they cease to have even minimal energy, or they have a seeming excess, to dispose of at once. They are all disabled people. They have become unbearably quarrelsome, or even dangerous at times, or self-neglectful, or even actively seeking death. If left to themselves some would wander about and die of exposure, others waste away, others destroy their own and others' property, or cause human harm. Families, friends and neighbours have always tried to restrain such people and care for them, but not everyone has a family to look after them, and those that do may pose severe problems of care.

To prevent wandering, persons 'of unsound mind' may be locked in or chained up. If they excrete carelessly about the house or attack the furniture they may be banished to an outhouse and sleep on straw on the floor, which is easier to clean up. Simply to have to live day after day with someone who is very depressed, or whose memory is impaired and who follows you everywhere all day for fear of losing touch, is emotionally draining. Such a person cannot be left alone, yet all relatives may need to be out at work. Except in very undeveloped countries or places where distances are great and families isolated, community aids develop to help with a lunatic. A village may create a temporary cell for the mad person, a monastery take in mad lodgers, private enterprise open madhouses or mental homes which make a profit out of taking in mad people, or the state uses prisons, workhouses, or concentration camps as repositories for the mentally disabled.

Concepts

'Madness' is a lay word, a social concept, not a medical one. The lunatic is judged to be mad by those around him, comparing his behaviour with the norm for that society. 'Mental illness', on the other hand, is independent of the environment (which may modify its manifestations, however); it is a disorder of function in the mind/brain, always a disability of some kind, a limitation on human free will. As a disorder it may not produce any social disharmony, or qualify as madness and therefore for compulsory treatment, although the doctor can recognise the malfunction by observation or a special test. So mental illness is commoner than 'madness', and some varieties would not be sent to an asylum.

Ideas about the nature of mental illness have changed over the centuries. In the past some 'madmen' have been regarded as possessed by spirits or devils, or in league with the Devil; or on the other hand as the chosen of God to experience and know matters hidden from the rest of us. Or madness has been seen as a malfunctioning, as when one is 'out of his senses' either for reasons unknown or following some devastating emotional experience, such as the deaths of all one's family. Because a mentally ill person shows alterations in behaviour which impinge on and provoke responses from those around him, the mad behaviour one observes is the fruit of the interaction between the individual and local society. This can be seen as starting in some abnormality in the individual, but it is possible to take the alternative view, that the individual's 'madness' is a response to the particular (persecutory, restrictive, rejecting) treatment he has received from family, neighbours, workmates, or bosses. However, if one meets a series of such individual sufferers it becomes apparent that they are not alike in their situations. In a few the social environment may play a very big part, in others there is a demonstrable physical illness which makes them abnormal, in yet others there are all kinds of combination of internal individual factors and external social ones. Naive analysis into black or white, or any other simple dichotomy such as mentally caused or physically caused, does not match the complexities of real life.

Sociologists and some non-medical historians have equated 'madness' with 'deviance'. This is a word which rather easily acquires more meaning than simply (statistical) difference from the norm. It may have moral or political overtones, implying sexual tastes or practices that many people disapprove of, or political views that are unacceptable to a majority, or even delinquency. Mentally ill people are deviant to the extent that they are not normal, but this is not moral or political deviance, and is indeed not what most distinguishes them. One can be more specific instead of referring to them as deviant in general. The distortion of the sense of reality, the excess or absence of emotion, the disturbance of common-sense thinking and sometimes of memory, the abnormal perceptions – these are the forms of difference from the ordinary man and woman. It is these distortions that may prevent a person coping with the world as it is and lead to a need for help. It is these distortions that can conceal from sufferers any awareness of their failure to cope, so that their judgement about themselves is no longer reliable, and compulsory treatment may be necessary to save them from themselves.

Why stop someone from committing suicide? There is a social answer and a personal answer. The first is that an individual is also almost invariably a member of a family and of a community and has certain duties towards both. Does a parent have the right to abandon a child by killing himself or herself? Has a highly trained or experienced person who normally contributes skilled work to the community no obligation to that community to continue contributing? Be that as it may, most suicide attempters caught in time are afterwards glad to be still alive, and do not try again the minute they are free to do so. Sometimes the act of rescue seems to be enough to finish the urge to die, at other times the urge goes only when psychiatric treatment has been given. The fact is, except when ill, most people do not want to die. Compulsion to live is justified by the return of the wish to live. Should we let the suicidal die?

Mentally ill people cannot perceive their deviance while they are ill, but they can recognise it later, when they have recovered, and are then often grateful to have been forced to have the treatment which has 'normalised' them. When should people be compelled to have treatment? How do we ensure that only those carefully defined as needing such treatment get it, and the compulsion does not spread to others who are socially or politically out of favour? These questions have in England been answered differently in 1890 from 1845, and changed again in 1930, 1959, and 1983.

Notes

For accounts of the management of the mad in other countries, see:

GIEL, R. & VAN LUIJK, J. N. (1969) Psychiatric morbidity in a small Ethiopian town. *British Journal of Psychiatry*, **115**, 149–162.
WESTERMEYER, J. & KROLL, J. (1978) Violence and mental illness in a peasant society (Laos). *British Journal of Psychiatry*, **133**, 529–541.

For a recent account of the symptoms and outcome of 'madness', see a textbook such as:

MAYER-GROSS, W., SLATER, E. & ROTH, M. (1960) *Clinical Psychiatry* (3rd edn). London: Cassell.

For descriptions of inhumane care of the mad, see:

JONES, K. (1972) *A History of the Mental Health Services*, pp. 56, 82–104. London: Routledge.

2 Why build an asylum?

The Buckingham County Pauper Lunatic Asylum was built because Parliament said it must. Part of the Lunatics Act (8 and 9 Vict.c.100) which received the Royal Assent on 8 August 1845 said that every county in England and Wales must build an asylum within three years. The county magistrates, through their meeting in Quarter Sessions, were to build it, and to find the money to do so by raising a local (county) rate. No money would come from central government. A committee of magistrates would be responsible for running the asylum and the annual costs would be divided among the parishes from which the patients came, in proportion to their lengths of stay in the asylum and their numbers. Although it was envisaged that the asylum might take private patients (and in fact from time to time it did so, when their families paid the weekly charges for board, lodging and medical care, etc.), the majority of those admitted would be kept without charge, and society, through the parish rates, provide for them. The asylum was not a charity, nor a profit-making institution, but a communal facility. As it became a hospital, if it was not one at first, it represented a first attempt at a community medical service, albeit of a specialised kind, and so may be seen as a forerunner of the National Health Service with its free hospitals of all kinds.

The magistrates may have seemed suitable people to create and run asylums because they were part of the legal system, and would be expected to show concern to avoid the risks of wrongful imprisonment or physical assault on patients, which had so often created unhappy scandals in previous private and public institutions. But they were also a part of the local government of the period, when the country gentlemen and the country clergy, with certain locally appointed officers, kept the peace and provided the social services. They had a great deal of autonomy, as will appear later in these pages. The government in London supplied what were in effect books of instructions on how to build and run asylums, and they vetted the plans for new buildings in a general way. The Commissioners in Lunacy with their staff in London provided regular inspections once or twice a year and a stream of advice, but the control was advisory only and the magistrates could more or less do as they liked. It was pure local government, because all the money was local.

The Lunatics Act 1845 was only one of many acts passed by Parliament for the better care for the mad. A glance at Table 2.1 shows that an astonishing amount of Parliamentary time was spent on this subject in the 19th century, and this raises two distinct questions. Why had England seemingly got along quite well for centuries without officially bothering about the mad, and then from 1800 made it a topic of the day? And why, from all the bother, did the county asylum emerge as a large part of the official solution to the problem? The answers to both questions are inevitably complex. To the first, demography gives a partial answer: the population began to expand and to live longer, and in consequence, insofar as the mad were a constant fraction of the population, there were more of them about. At the same time the agricultural revolution of the 18th century and the industrial revolution which followed it combined to break up the old ways of rural life and to create new cities, where madness became more visible.

TABLE 2.1
Statutes relating to the care of the mentally ill, 1744–1983

Year	Act
1744	Act for Regulating Private Madhouses
1808	County Asylums Act (amended 1811, 1815, 1819)
1828	County Asylums Act
	Madhouse Act
1832	Lunatics Act
1834	*Poor Law Amendment Act*
1842	Lunatic Asylums Act
1845	Lunatics Act
	Lunatic Asylums and Pauper Lunatics Act
1853	Lunacy Regulations Act
	Lunatics Care and Treatment Amendment Act
	Lunatic Asylums Amendment Act
1862	Lunatics Law Amendment Act
1886	Idiots Act[1]
1889	Lunatics Law Amendment Act
1890	**Lunacy (Consolidation) Act**
1891	Lunacy Act
1899	Elementary Education (Defective & Epileptic Children) Act[1]
1913	Mental Deficiency Act[1]
1914	Elementary Education (Defective & Epileptic Children) Act
1927	Mental Deficiency Act[1]
1929	*Local Government Act*
1930	Mental Treatment Act
1946	**National Health Service Act**
1959	**Mental Health Act**
1983	**Mental Health Act**

Bold type denotes particular importance; Acts of tangential importance to this field are in italic.
Note also Poor Law Act 1601; Vagrancy Acts of 1567, 1714, 1744.
1. Laws dealing specifically with those mentally handicapped, retarded or deficient from birth as distinct from those of normal growth and development who became mentally *ill* when adult.

The old ways of dealing with the mad broke down, and new, unsatisfactory ways grew up spontaneously and by their unsatisfactoriness provoked legal control.

To the second question, the previous history of local government in England is a partial explanation, but so is the contemporary state of the Christian religion and beliefs, and the stage of development of the sciences relating to man. The county asylum was an obvious development of what had gone before, but it also represented a view of human nature and of man's relationship to man, just as a monastery, a prison, a boarding school or a regular army do. It will be interesting to look at these matters in more detail.

Growth of the population

Although the first government census of the inhabitants of England and Wales took place in 1801, a fair idea of the earlier size of the nations and of the principal cities can be gained from study of a great variety of parish and municipal records of birth and marriage, tax returns, and so forth. We know that since Roman times the total population has fluctuated probably between one and five million, sometimes cut down by the great epidemics (such as the Black Death (1348–50) and the Great Plague (1664–67) or the ravages of syphilis (15th century), smallpox and perhaps influenza), sometimes static, sometimes increasing again. One such increase began about 1760, but differed from its predecessors in being long-sustained, in fact lasting to the present day: we are at the moment about 50 million strong. This increase has varied in rate: in the mid 19th century the population was growing by about two million every ten years, but at the end of the century it rose by three and a half million each decade, and after 1911 dropped back again to around two million.

Buckinghamshire shared in this population growth, but to a lesser extent until recently (Table 2.2). In the century to 1901 the national population grew fourfold, but that of Bucks only doubled; meanwhile London grew eightfold, maintaining its position of always being about ten times the size of any other city. When the Bucks County Pauper Lunatic Asylum opened at the half century, Bucks had about 143 000 people: by 1961 St John's served a population about three times greater. If we assume that there is a constant rate of madness in the population as a whole (of about one or two per thousand) then the number of lunatics must have increased fourfold during the 19th century (eightfold in London), and even doubled in Bucks.

But madness does not strike equally at all ages, and of course it is not an entity anyway, but a collection of different conditions which vary individually in incidence from time to time. Nevertheless people are much more likely to develop one of these conditions in middle age, or later, while children very rarely do, and the growth of the population in the last 180 years

TABLE 2.2
National and county population changes, 1801–1981

Area	Population		
	1801	*1901*	*1981*
Total population, England and Wales	8 million	32 million	50 million
Buckinghamshire	108 000	196 000	568 000
London	800 000	6.5 million	

Ignores minor changes in geographical boundaries.

has occurred largely because people live much longer than they used to. The expectation of life was about 45 years in 1850, and it is now over 70; in Roman times, to judge by the tombstone inscriptions in Roman cemeteries, it cannot have been much more than 30.

While the Bucks population trebled between 1851 and 1961 (Table 2.3), the over-60s increased five times and girls under 20 only doubled in number: they were about a quarter of the population in 1851, but only an eighth in 1961. This change in the age structure of the population again points to increases in the number of the mad beyond that expected from simply counting total heads in the population.

Why has the population grown in this way since 1760? Perhaps better nutrition in the late 18th century increased fertility – the likelihood that an act of intercourse would result in pregnancy or a decrease in the likelihood of spontaneous abortion, or both. Changes in the age of marriage (influenced by economic factors) and in the efficiency and practice of contraception are important. Above all, apart from the disappearance of fatal diseases such as plague and smallpox, the great improvement of food supplies, after the agricultural revolution of the 18th century and the industrial revolution of the 19th, has not only supported a tenfold increase in mouths to be fed but has increased bodily resistance to disease and reduced mortality at all ages, particularly among infants and young children where it used to be so high. London's Foundling Hospital was opened in 1741 to take care of the many newborn babies being abandoned in the streets, and it is interesting that out of 14 934 babies under two months old when admitted in the hospital's early years, 10 389 failed to reach a year old. This no longer happens.

TABLE 2.3
Age structure of the Buckinghamshire population, 1851 and 1961

	1851	*1961*
Total population	143 000	488 000
Number aged over 60	5 900	30 300
Girls aged under 20	32 900	64 000

The social background to the emergence of the county asylums

The agricultural revolution reduced employment on the land. The industrial revolution offered jobs in the cities. They were often completely new jobs because of the new technology – many thousands for instance were involved in building the railways, making and servicing the engines and carriages, and running the trains; this led to the creation of new towns such as Wolverton (Bucks), Swindon, and Crewe. Thus many thousands of people flooded into the towns from the country, helped by the better transport facilities – the Oxford Canal (1774–90), the Grand Junction Canal with branch to Aylesbury (1793–1805), the London to Birmingham railway via Wolverton in north-east Bucks (1838), and the Great Western railway route from Paddington to Bristol via Slough in south Bucks (also 1838).

The existence of railways encouraged much more movement about the country. In 1851, for instance, an inhabitant of Buckingham could take a day excursion (56 miles each way) to the Great Exhibition in Hyde Park, London. Aylesbury, about 30 miles from London, and previously a five-hour journey by horse and carriage, eventually became a one-hour journey by train. The mentally ill could wander further afield, and became more noticeable in strange surroundings. The shift to the city meant much less space to live in, and neighbours on all sides were more aware of what each other were doing. The mentally ill were likely to be surrounded by strangers, while relatives and former friends were still in the country or gone elsewhere. The old supports of family, village, church and squire were gone, yet in the city people were forced into physically closer relationships at work and at home. The mad were less hidden, more of a communal nuisance.

It is not surprising therefore that charity hospitals for the mentally ill began to appear in the growing cities. For centuries London had had the only mental hospital in the whole country, Bethlem, with room for only 30 patients before 1676. It had begun as a religious charity, taken by the Crown at the dissolution of the monasteries and handed to the City of London. In the 18th century the general hospital newly founded by Mr Guy (1725) explicitly included a wing for the chronically disabled, including the mentally ill, and in 1751 a whole new specialist hospital, St Luke's, was opened by public subscription. Manchester and Liverpool, the two largest and most rapidly growing industrial cities after London, opened similar charitable mental hospitals in 1763 and 1797 respectively, as offshoots of their new general infirmaries. These mental hospitals took patients for modest fees, and some poor people for nothing. Some cities that were old cultural centres also started charitable mental hospitals – York (population 16 000 in 1801, a fifth that of Manchester) gained the famous Retreat in 1796 and Oxford (population under 12 000 in 1801) had from 1826 the Warneford Hospital as an offshoot of the Radcliffe Infirmary (Table 2.4).

Apart from these rather few public-spirited provisions for the mad, the 18th century saw an increase in the number of private madhouses, small

TABLE 2.4
Some English public institutions for the mad, to 1853

Year	Institution
1377	Priory of St Mary of Bethlehem (founded 1247), in London. Taken by the Crown at the Dissolution, from 1546 owned by the City of London and became Bethlem Royal Hospital, first situated at the present site of Liverpool Street; 1676 new building at Moorfields, 1816 new building at St George's Fields, Vauxhall, 1928, new building at Beckenham, Kent
1713	Bethel at Norwich
1725	Thomas Guy provides wing in his new hospital for chronic patients (including lunatics)
1751	St Luke's Asylum, London, the first subscription hospital
1766	Manchester Lunatic Hospital: an offshoot of the Infirmary
1765	Hospital for lunatics for the counties of Northumberland, Newcastle and Durham
1777	York asylum
1796	The Retreat, York
1797	Liverpool asylum
1811	County asylum, Nottingham
1812	County asylum, Bedford
1814	County asylum, Thorpe (Norfolk)
1816	Lancaster asylum
1818	Stafford and Wakefield asylums
1823	Gloucester asylum
1829	Bodmin (Cornwall) and Lincoln asylums
1828–42	Chester, Dorset, Kent, Middlesex, Norfolk, Suffolk, Surrey and Leicester asylums
1838	Northampton asylum
1846	Oxford (Littlemore) (Warneford, an offshoot of the Radcliffe Infirmary, was opened in 1826)
1853	County asylum, Buckinghamshire

individually owned establishments run for profit. They were dotted about the countryside: a clergyman might decide to take a few patients in his large vicarage or a country house be converted to take 10–20 patients. These enterprises were often quite short lived, and before the beginnings of legal control through licensing in 1774, there is almost no information about them, except for scandals of wrongful confinement or inhumane treatment. A few, however, continued under successive generations of the same family of owners, those at Hook Norton and Witney in Oxfordshire for instance, or Ticehurst in Kent.

In the first half of the 19th century they grew and multiplied, and some began to take in the poor as well. A census taken on 1 January 1847 said there were 77 licensed private houses or private asylums in England and Wales housing 3574 private patients and 9652 paupers (paid for by their parishes), and at this time the private enterprise asylums provided for more cases than did the public institutions. The government was quite prepared to make use of them. In 1814, for instance, it was noted (because of some scandal there) that a private madhouse in Hoxton in addition to its fee-paying patients was housing 14 mentally ill officers and 136 mentally ill seamen from the Royal Navy, among a force of 486 'pauper' patients.

Growing industrialisation and urbanisation brought the mad to public attention. People's increasing wealth from the growing empire in India, the West Indies and the Americas helped to pay the fees of private madhouses. George III's episodes of madness in 1788–89, 1801, 1804, 1805, and 1810 publicised and made almost respectable the existence of madness. Murders or attempted murders by lunatics (1800 Hadfield shot at George III, Drury Lane Theatre; 1812 Bellingham killed the Prime Minister Spencer Perceval; 1840 Oxford shot at Queen Victoria on Constitution Hill; 1843 McNaughton killed Drummond in mistake for the Prime Minister Sir Robert Peel) were public reminders of its importance. Then the population explosion and longer lives sent the number of lunatics leaping. Government had to do something about it. Providing evenly for all, across the country, what was hitherto available spasmodically and chiefly to the rich, came to be the basis of it.

Buckinghamshire in the 1830s

Although chair-making was an old-established industry, and lace-making and glove-making cottage occupations, Buckinghamshire was essentially a farming county. As such its population suffered two setbacks before 1838, the critical year in which the railways came and began to improve the situation. The later setback was the great drop in corn prices after the end of the Napoleonic Wars (1815), which threatened farmers with bankruptcy and threw many labourers out of work; the earlier one was the land enclosures which took away the small man's common land on which he could graze a cow or grow vegetables. It is true that the enclosures increased agricultural efficiency, so that much more food was to be produced and a larger national population supported, but they took away the poor villager's insurance against hard times, and financial compensation for his loss of common rights was no substitute. The Bledlow affair of 1834 is illustrative.

In this Chiltern village there were then 156 agricultural labourers aged over 20, and because of the slump wages were very low, 2s 6d per week for single men and 7s 0d per week for married men, at a time when five loaves of bread cost 4s 0d, rent was 1s 2d, and shoes were 15s 0d a pair. In fact the parish was having to find an average of nearly £36 per week (at 20s to the £1) for poor relief, and many families were close to starvation. Thirty-two of the unemployed men got together and appealed to the West Wycombe magistrates (their local authority) for the loan of land on which to grow potatoes. This was refused. They then appealed to the newly appointed Poor Law Commissioners in London, who sent an investigator to report. The unemployed were offered jobs in the new mills in Lancashire, and in early 1835 a number of families were despatched there with all their goods and chattels by canal boat at parish expense, and 83 people found jobs. The hours were very long, and the wages low by Lancashire standards, but at anything from 10s 0d to 28s 0d per week they represented an improvement for the Bledlow men.

With the advent of the railways, Bucks was brought within easy distance of London and it became a big supplier of agricultural and horticultural produce to the growing city. Bucks people could more easily go to London to work, and domestic service in the city was employing increasing numbers. This easy travel took more and more people from their birthplace, their home parish, into foreign surroundings, where they might fall ill. It also brought more strangers into Bucks, both those working on the railways and those passing through, like the butler who stepped off the Holyhead–London train at Leighton Buzzard and was found wandering in delirium on the platform. He recovered in a few days in the Bucks County Asylum and was then able to explain that he had been in an Irish country house but dismissed for heavy drinking, and was on his way home to London when delirium tremens struck him.

The way that people were shifting about, even in a rural county like Bucks, is shown by the increasing population of its towns, even between 1801 and 1851 (Table 2.5). All this movement played havoc with the social services of the time, which for centuries had been based on the idea that each parish cared only for its own native poor, sick, or disabled.

At one time each parish had to send in an annual return of the number of 'lunatics' it was paying something for, whether they were dangerous, and where they were. The returns for 1838 in the County Record Office, known to be missing many cases, reported 22 lunatics and 32 idiots among 100 parishes. Some of the lunatics were confined at home, some were allowed full liberty, and some were away in asylums. Thus Sophia Pickforth, aged 40, was shut up at Pitstone and the parish paid 5s per week for her; Elizabeth Foxley, ill for 27 years, was in a cottage with her daughter and received 5s; Sarah Green age 64 had been in Stafford Lunatic Asylum for the previous five years; and Elizabeth Harris, aged 40, was in the White House, Bethnal Green, in London at a cost of 10s per week. Others were "with friends", or "at Mrs Allen's", or "with mother" or in the workhouse, which cost only 3s per week.

In 1838 Denham Park was opened as a private licensed house for up to 17 paying patients by Sir William Charles Ellis and Edward Hornor, but only

TABLE 2.5
Size of some towns in Buckinghamshire

	1801	1851	1901	1961
County population	108 000	143 000	196 000	488 000
Aylesbury	3186	6081	9099	27 923
Buckingham	2605	4020	3152	
High Wycombe	4248	7179	19 282	49 981
Amersham	2314	3662	3209	56 005
Chesham	3969	6098	9005	
Bletchley	1038	1544	4269	
Wolverton	238	2070		

Wolverton and Bletchley were railway towns.

one out of over 50 patients in six years, a farmer's wife, came from Bucks, the others giving addresses in Durham, Stamford, Yorkshire, Kent, Saffron Walden, and of course London (including a tavern-keeper from Blackwall). A few Bucks residents previously had gone to the Warneford Hospital in Oxford, opened in 1826. The report of the Metropolitan Commissioners in Lunacy to the Lord Chancellor in 1844 surveying nationally the public and private facilities for the mad noted that Buckinghamshire was one of 11 counties without any private or public asylums whatsoever, yet according to their estimate there were 147 potential patients in the county, a number of them in the local workhouses. In 1854 they recorded 11 in Amersham, and 15 in Newport Pagnell workhouses, for instance, and similar numbers in the four other county institutions.

Caring for the poor and disabled

At least since 1601 social services were based on the parish. Each parish was responsible for its own native sons and daughters only, and it was assumed that there would be few people away from home, and even fewer travellers or immigrants who would be in need of care. If any such appeared in a parish, the officers were supposed to identify their homes and send them back there for care, and the sending might involve transfer from one parish to another in sequence across the country until the person reached home. This could be cumbersome and difficult to arrange at best, and broke down altogether if the sufferer had no home, or could or would not reveal it, or if the parish he named as home refused to acknowledge him. Travelling pedlars, strolling players, wandering scholars, the unemployed in search of work, men who had abandoned their wives and families to the parish, vagrants, rogues, gypsies, discharged soldiers, beggars, the mentally ill . . . most of those on the road in the 17th and early 18th century were regarded with suspicion by the authorities.

The second principle in succouring the poor and disabled was the provision of money ('outdoor relief'), not accommodation, which of course fitted in with the idea that those to be helped already had homes of some sort in the parish. As the number of travellers on the road increased in the 18th century, the problem of accommodating them grew, and they were likely to find themselves deposited in a gaol (a 'house of correction') or a bridewell, or a workhouse. The gaol was primarily a place of punishment for those who had broken the law, and the prisoner (or his family) were expected to pay for his keep there. In a bridewell or debtors' prison, the prisoner lived free, but under very poor condition because the manager of the bridewell received an annual sum from the county to cover all costs – salaries of assistants, maintenance of the building, his own salary and profits, and the food and care of the prisoners (which naturally came last, particularly as there was no supervision). Workhouses grew up as places where the itinerant unemployed, people who could not afford a home, the disabled, the chronic sick, the idiots, imbeciles, and mad, could be taken in off the streets and given some kind of manual labour to do in exchange for their keep; the conditions were very poor in order to drive the inmates out, to proper jobs. A growing proportion of them were incapable of this, and simply rotted in the workhouse until the poor food, poor hygiene, poor ventilation, overcrowding, and lack of medical or surgical care led to dysentery, typhoid, pneumonia or tuberculosis, and death.

The good side of the parish system of relief is seen in the case of George Monk of Chalfont St Giles, a village 23 miles from London in the south of Bucks. The details come from the vestry accounts. He became mentally ill in 1739, and in June was taken on horseback for admission to Bethlem Hospital in London, then at Moorfields. The parish had to pay the hospital "to the committee at entry, 10s 6d, to the steward for bedding £1-14-0, for bonds and clerk £1-1-0, and for the certificate 4s 0d". He was discharged better after about four months in October of the same year, and brought home "with the looker-after and porter, 4s 0d. Expenses with him, my horse and theirs, and on the Roade, 15s 0d". Meanwhile his wife Ann Monk had been provided with a monthly pension of 4s 0d.

For a time he was well, but he broke down again in 1740, and subsequently was ill in 1749–50 and 1754. On these occasions he did not go back to London but a special 'cage', or one-person hospital, was constructed for him near the church, and he was looked after there, as shown by various payments: January 1750, "paid Jane Garman for looking after George Monk 2s 0d. 1750 paid Dame Field for looking after George Monk 2s 0d, 1 truss of straw for G M, 0s 6d"; and in May 1754 "paid for lock and chaine for George Monk 5s 6d". Thus the village out of its local funds provided medical and nursing care, and financial and social support to the patient's wife and 'girl'. Other 18th-century villages did likewise. Porter in *Mind Forg'd Manacles* (1987, p. 120) mentions Cheriton Fitzpaine in Devon where in 1723 a villager ran wild, was captured, brought back and cleaned up and then 'warded' for payment by the parish with a clergyman-doctor while maintenance was paid to the patient's wife and children.

This kind of rather personal care was hardly possible in a big town, but in any case was unlikely to be offered to a newcomer. The bad side of the alternatives of care in workhouse or private madhouse can be illustrated by two descriptions quoted by Kathleen Jones in *A History of the Mental Health Services* (1972) and which will do for many experiences quoted in official reports. In a Cornish workhouse in 1815 two women were found chained to a damp stone floor in separate cells, one of which was dark and airless. One had a little dirty straw to lie on; it had been there for weeks, she was not allowed to wash herself, and the cell was filled with excrement. She had apparently been confined many months, summer and winter, because she was troublesome (not violent at all) and kept wandering about the country and people complained about her.

In a private madhouse owned by Warburton in London, pauper patients were sometimes (as noted at public inquiries in 1816 and again in 1827) kept in cribs, wooden cases filled with straw, where they lay naked covered with a blanket. The unclean patients were put in the cribs at 3 p.m., their arms and legs chained, and left till 9 a.m. next day. At weekends they spent from 3 p.m. Saturday to 9 a.m. Monday in the crib, and their arms partially released so they could eat when food was brought. On Mondays they were mopped down with cold water in the yard to get the excrement off them. Their straw sometimes contained maggots.

No proper records were kept, and some inmates went completely unrecorded till they died: no reason why they came in, who had arranged it, what treatment they had, or anything about their injuries and illnesses was recorded. Between 1744 (the Act for Regulating Private Madhouses) and 1845 (the Lunatics Act, and the subsidiary Act to erect and run county asylums), government proceeded by slow stages, beginning with attempts to inspect some of the places where lunatics were kept, widening the inspection and introducing penalties for abuses, requiring madhouses to be licensed and keep registers of those admitted and discharged, laying down procedures to be fulfilled if someone was to be sent to a madhouse or asylum. Each step in tightening the screw of inspection and control met opposition, sometimes prolonged, but the long-renewed experiences of abuses, at first wrongful detention and later grossly inhumane and indifferent care, served to strengthen the push for reform. The County Asylum Act 1808 was one landmark, with its specification of what a public asylum should be and do: it permitted counties to build asylums if they so wished, but over the next 20 years only nine did so. The two Acts of 1828 were a second landmark, providing for regular inspections by special commissioners in London, and by visiting Justices of the Peace elsewhere reporting to the Home Secretary, and requiring the keeping of records and statistics and the provision of medical attendance at all private madhouses and subscription hospitals, and all county asylums.

The Acts of 1845 strengthened the earlier provisions, and made the building of county asylums compulsory. The Special London (Metropolitan) Commissioners were reorganised into a national inspectorate and controlling body, the Lunacy Commission, under the Lord Chancellor. There were five lay commissioners, unpaid, one acting as chairman, and three doctors and three lawyers paid full-time, who carried out the regular inspections, the whole backed by a small secretariat. They were to license all London madhouses, and to receive copies of provincial licenses issued by local magistrates; and they were to issue formal reports on their work to the Lord Chancellor three times a year. Their main function, however, was inspection – all hospitals, all licensed houses, all gaols and workhouses, and even, in certain circumstances, single lunatics. They could inspect all buildings and outhouses by day or by night, see all patients under restraint, and see all the prescribed records. In addition they became a source of advice to all those running asylums.

There was a certain parallel in this organisation for mental illness to that earlier established by the Poor Law Amendment Act 1834 for the unemployed and homeless. A central Poor Law Commission ruled in London, while around the country parishes were grouped together in unions, which had to build and maintain workhouses to lodge the homeless, shiftless, penniless and other social rejects.

In the Lunatics Act 1845 the certificates required as safeguards against wrongful detention differed somewhat for private and for pauper patients. For the former, someone had to request that the patient be admitted (to madhouse or asylum), giving a rudimentary medical and social history, and explaining who the requester was (occupation, address, relationship to patient). The request had to be accompanied by certificates from two separate doctors stating why they thought the patient should be confined. For the pauper, the request to admit was signed by a JP or clergyman of the parish, and also by the relieving officer or overseer of the poor. Thus the responsibility for determining compulsory admission to an asylum rested primarily with lay people, and if they did not request it, nothing happened. Thus lunatics would still remain at home if the family wished, and of course those seen as lunatics were only a part of all those people who were mentally ill.

The Act also required the keeping of record books: admission, diagnosis, ultimate fate, restraint, seclusion, injuries, violence, a medical case book, and a visitor's book. Various notices had to be sent to the Lunacy Commission and for the JPs.

A prime mover behind the 1845 Acts, and a force in the Lunacy Commission for the next 40 years, was Lord Ashley, later the seventh Lord Shaftesbury, already noted for his work in fighting for the abolition of slavery, and in seeking to improve the conditions of employment of children and women in mines and factories. He represented the spirit of Christian compassion, of care for others, the weak and the unfortunate, which was such a distinct strand in the outlook of many in Victorian society. For him the lunatic was a human being with a disability, a human soul with human rights, not some animal that needed to be chained up, or to be hectored and beaten and terrorised. Under his guidance the county pauper asylums aimed to be models of kindly care and treatment in good surroundings and with good food, a contrast to the workhouses, and for very many years this was the ethos.

Notes

Some sources for this chapter included:

CARTWRIGHT, F. F. (1977) *A Social History of Medicine.* London: Longman.
JONES, K. (1972) *A History of the Mental Health Services.* London: Routledge.
PARRY-JONES, W. L. (1971) *The Trade in Lunacy.* London: Routledge.

Papers in County Record Office (Denham Park etc.).

PORTER, R. (1987) *Mind Forg'd Manacles*. London: Athlone Press.

"Records of Bucks", XVIII, part 1 (1966) on George Monk.

"Records of Bucks", XVIII, part 4 (1969) on the Bledlow affair.

REED, M. (1979) *The Buckinghamshire Landscape*. London: Hodder & Stoughton.

Reports of decennial censuses, Aylesbury Reference Library.

II. Managing lunatics

3 A hotel in the country

The country gentlemen of Bucks who were the magistrates appointed at Quarter Sessions in 1846 to create a county asylum (see Table 3.1) can be excused for a certain lack of enthusiasm for the project. They were not sure of the need, in a rural county without a big city, and they resented the expense. They and their fellow ratepayers would have to foot the bills for land and buildings now, and for yearly maintenance ever after, even if the annual running costs came from the poor rate collected by the parish councils. Indeed, one of their first jobs was to reject appeals from ten areas of the county asking them not to comply with the 1845 Act. Their first plan was not to build it themselves but to join with a neighbour (Oxford, Northampton

TABLE 3.1

The 13 magistrates who planned the asylum

Christopher Tower (Chairman)
The Most Noble Richard Plantagenet Campbell, Marquis of Chandos
Right Honourable George, Lord Nugent
Sir Thomas Digby Aubrey
Sir Harry Verney[1]
Dr John Lee, LLD[2]
Thomas Raymond Barker[3]
Thomas Alexander Boswell
George Carrington, the Younger[4]
James Trevor Senior
Rev. George Chetwode
Rev. John Harrison
John Newman

The Clerk to the Committee was Mr Acton Tindal, the Clerk of the Peace and a leading solicitor in Aylesbury. Manor House, later to be Manor House Hospital, was built for him, and Tindal General Hospital named after him.
1. The brother-in-law of Florence Nightingale.
2. Later a president of the Royal Astronomical Society, helped to found the Royal Bucks Hospital, and was a noted reformer.
3. Chairman of Committee, 1857–65.
4. Chairman, Committee of Visitors, 1853–56.
Messrs Tower, Lee and Senior were also members of the Committee of Visitors for some years.

29

or Bedford) which already had an asylum and for a modest financial outlay gain the right to send Bucks lunatics there. But one was not willing, another was too small, and they felt that Bedford was too far for relatives to visit.

Land and water

Accordingly, when a year had gone by with the slow tempo of meetings at Quarter Sessions, they advertised for suitable land in the area of Aylesbury, the county town. Here a further delay loomed. They had no powers of compulsory purchase, and landowners seemed unwilling to sell to accommodate lunatics. A full advertisement in the three local papers, the *Bucks Herald*, *Bucks Gazette* and *Aylesbury News* and in the national *Times* in November and December of 1847 brought no response, and they started contacting possible vendors directly. Two members of the Magistrates' Committee offered sites, Lord Nugent near Winslow and Dr Lee near Bishopstone and Ford, but these were not approved.

A further advertisement a year later (Fig. 3.1) in the local papers produced about seven further offers which were also rejected. Finally, the

County of Buckingham.

THE Justices of the Peace for the County not having yet determined upon the selection of a site for a Pauper Lunatic Asylum, are desirous of receiving further Tenders from persons willing to offer land for sale for this purpose.

Twenty acres at least of Freehold Land, in a perfectly healthy situation, will be required, as central as possible to the mass of population in the County, and convenient and easy of access by public conveyances and for the supply of all necessary stores. An elevated and cheerful position is desirable, and the surrounding country should be undulating in its surface, and not near to any nuisances, such as steam engines, noisy trades, or offensive manufactures; nor surrounded, overlooked, or liable to be inconvenienced by the neighbourhood of public roads or footpaths. The site must possess the means of affording an ample supply of good water and facilities for obtaining a good system of drainage. A chalky, gravelly, or rocky subsoil is most desirable, but if a clayey subsoil only can be obtained, an elevated position is indispensable.

Applications, stating fully and clearly all the above particulars, and the price, are requested to be made to me on or before Monday, the 6th day of November next, in order that the same may be laid before the Committee appointed to superintend the erecting or providing of an Asylum for the Pauper Lunatics of this County, pursuant to the Act 8th and 9th Victoria, cap. 126.

ACTON TINDAL,
Clerk of the Peace for Bucks.

Aylesbury, 24th Oct., 1848.

Fig. 3.1. The advertisement for land upon which to build the asylum. The specification is that of the Commissioners

Reverend Joseph Bancroft Reade, vicar of Stone, offered some of his glebe land, good farming land enclosed in 1777, but he wanted more for it per acre than almost all the other offers had asked, and the Magistrates' Committee did not want to pay so much. In the end, however, they decided to take it, at £150 per acre, and to buy 20 acres, subject to the approval of the Bishop, the Commissioners in Lunacy and the Secretary of State (for Home Affairs), which was soon granted. It was a site four miles out of Aylesbury, to the south of the Aylesbury–Thame (Oxford) turnpike road, with a slight slope and southerly aspect to the Chiltern hills (Fig. 3.2).

The Commissioners in Lunacy recommended providing an acre for every 10 patients, so that 20 acres would accommodate 200 patients; they also held that an asylum should not be too big, and tried to set an upper limit of 250 beds so that it would not become impersonal. Up to this time most of the private and public institutions had in fact been smaller. Later, when the numbers of patients became larger, magistrates insisted on building much larger asylums rather than additional small ones, in order to save money, whatever the Commissioners might say. Of course it must be remembered

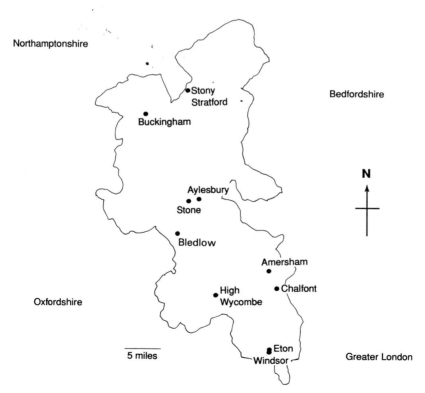

Fig. 3.2. A map of Buckinghamshire (modern Milton Keynes is by Stony Stratford)

that 200 beds would serve to treat more than 200 patients because, at least in 1850, it was envisaged that many patients would get better in a matter of months and be able to leave the asylum for good.

The problem for the Committee was how many to build for. In 1845 the annual return to the Bucks Clerk of the Peace from the various Bucks parishes had indicated about 92 lunatics and 93 idiots being paid for out of parish funds, those at home or with friends at the rate of about three shillings a week, those in private or public asylums at nine or ten shillings. In 1850 they heard of 153 lunatics – 10 in a public asylum in some other county, 108 in private asylums or licensed houses, 26 in union workhouses (a very unreliable count here) and 9 with friends or elsewhere. Sixty-three per cent of these Bucks folk were women. The Committee varied from time to time in the size they planned for, but by 1850 it was 100 for each sex, with the proviso that the asylum could be easily expanded by 50.

In general the land the magistrates had bought conformed well with the recommendations of the Commissioners in Lunacy in London, but in one important respect it fell short. It did not seem likely to provide a water supply of 40 gallons per head per day. Such a quantity of water no doubt seemed quite excessive and unnecessary to the Committee. A consultant civil engineer, J. Neville Warren, confirmed them in their view. He pointed out that at that time the water consumption in London, including industrial as well as domestic use, worked out at 11 ¾ gallons per inhabitant per day, so 40 gallons was obviously nonsense.

The Commissioners in Lunacy knew better, because of the very careful surveys of private and public asylums, old and new, they had made. The water supply of course covers not only the patients but the resident staff, not to speak of the horses in the stables, the animals on the farm, the plants in the gardens. But an asylum needed an unusually large amount of water because of the quantity of laundry and the need for frequent washing of floors and furniture, as some psychiatric patients are deficient in personal hygiene.

The mistaken ideas about water interfered with the asylum's work in the early years, and caused the Committee much concern and the ratepayers eventually considerable extra expense.

Building

With the site of the asylum settled, seven architects of repute, including G. G. Scott, were invited to submit plans for the building. Four of them responded, and in September 1849 Messrs Wyatt and Brandon of London were selected. The firm had been responsible for numerous churches in Wiltshire, the assize court at Devizes, and was then building the Wiltshire County Asylum (opened in 1851) at Roundway. David Brandon in fact became the responsible architect for the Buckinghamshire asylum, and for the extensions in 1864 and 1868. He was then 37, and was later noted for building large Victorian country houses.

His design was severely limited by the Commissioners' requirements, which were specified in some detail. They were anxious to get as much light, sunshine and air into the building as possible (hence a radial plan was unacceptable) and were very concerned about good ventilation and adequate heating. They specified single bedrooms for one-third of the patients, and dormitories of up to 12 beds for the others, as both more friendly and easier to supervise. Single rooms were to be 9 by 6½ feet by 11 to 12½ feet high; rather less space per patient (48 square feet of floor, 576 cubic feet of air) in the dormitories. The day rooms should each have an open fireplace (a fire is cheerful) and allow at least 10 square feet of floor per patient, and be easily accessible from a kitchen. Long galleries, such as are seen in some old country houses, were to be provided so that patients would have somewhere to walk, exercise, and play games when the weather was too wet or cold for them to go outside.

There should be enough separate wards to keep the violent and noisy away from the tranquil: aged and infirm, epileptic, and incontinent should be separable. There should be a chapel big enough to hold at least half the patients at once for divine service. Most importantly, males and females were to be kept completely segregated, each sex in its own buildings, staff as well as patients. There was such a fear of sex that it was laid down that one of the matron's jobs was to chaperone all female staff whenever they were to be spoken to by the Superintendent; and even in 1892 the inspecting Commissioners criticised the fact that some male and female patients could meet during the day while at work helping in the laundry or kitchens.

Other requirements for the design came from the Magistrates' Committee. They wanted most of the sleeping accommodation upstairs, requiring a two-level building, and the possibility of expanding it easily later. They were greatly concerned about the risks of fire, and wanted to avoid the use of wood in construction where possible. Although Mr Wyatt assured them it was quite unnecessary, they opted for iron window frames (which did not fit well and let in the rain) and iron ceilings, which added over £700 to the cost, and with the concrete floors added to the weight the walls had to carry. They had all the fireplaces blocked up in rooms used by patients, presumably fearing arsonists, or epileptics falling into a fire during a fit, and this threw a burden on the ventilation and heating system. Normally warm air in a room rises in the chimney to the outside and fresh colder air is drawn in through windows and ventilators and through doorways or under doors. They did not want windows to open much either, for fear of patients jumping out to escape or commit suicide. But air conditioning and central heating were then both in their infancy. It is no surprise, though unfortunate, that the chosen method, Mr Price's patent system, though already installed in Colney Hatch (now Friern Barnet), a big Middlesex asylum, proved a very considerable failure and occasioned much work and modification.

The system was essentially a hot-air system, the air heated by hot water from the same boilers which supplied the baths and wash-basins. At the south-east and south-west front corners of the building stood two towers, at the base of which a boiler produced hot water and warm air which ran along flues under the galleries. This was supposed to warm the rooms above them. Ventilators near the tops of the rooms opened into horizontal flues which eventually communicated with the up-draught in the tower. It was found that the system did not warm the wards very well, especially those at some distance from the boilers, and on expert study proved to be incapable of doing its job (no proper physical calculations of heat transfer had been made). The boilers were far too small, and inefficient, the distances the hot water and hot air were to travel were far too great, and the number of pipes and flues inadequate. Chanter's patent stoves had to be placed in the wards, and the blocked fireplaces opened up; the boilers had to be replaced by much bigger, modern ones, with bigger surfaces against the burning coal.

It is interesting to see what the big new country houses of the rich were like at the mid-century. Water closets were commonly fitted, but wash-basins rarely and fixed baths often not at all. Basins filled from a jug and hip baths carried by servants into bedrooms as needed were much more usual. Central heating, first by ducted hot air, later by hot water circulating in pipes and radiators, was beginning to come in, and Mentmore, built not far from Aylesbury for a Rothschild in 1852, was one of the first houses to have a hot water system; steam heating came after the Victorian period. Lighting by gas as opposed to oil-lamps or candles was rare outside towns (Aylesbury had a town gas-works from 1834): it posed ventilation problems and was not very efficient until the invention of the incandescent mantle about 1880.

Brandon designed the asylum like a country house, to a standard of technical comfort above that most patients would have known in their own homes, with their candles and oil-lamps, garden earth privies, yard taps and communal pumps. For each sex of 100 patients there were four bathrooms, with a bath and three to five wash-basins in each, and 12 water closets. There were 168 gas-lamps, supplied from a gas-works constructed at the south-west corner of the estate (see p. 69). There were central hot water, heating and ventilation systems, with boiler houses. There were long galleries for indoor exercise. There were approximately 12 acres for outdoor walks, growing vegetables, and keeping farm animals; and coach houses and stables for up to six horses. (Since there was no ambulance service, and of course no telephone or telegraph, communications and the transfer of patients to and from the asylum depended on horses.) Coal, stores, and food came from Aylesbury, the county town four miles away, by horse transport.

The plan of the building (Figs 3.3, 3.4) was a central administration block on a north–south axis, separating parallel 'L'-shaped long blocks for men on the west and women on the east. In both cases the foot of the 'L' faced south, the two feet meeting and fusing with the Superintendent's house (and matron's quarters) in the centre of the southern facade. Behind (to the north of this house) were the kitchens and foodstores with a chapel above (with three separate entrances, one for staff, and one each for male and female patients). Further north, the administration block had examination rooms for new patients, rooms for visitors (who were not allowed in the wards) and the steward's (lay administrator's) office, bedroom and parlour.

At the northern tip of the women's wards was the laundry; at a similar position on the male side carpenter's, tailor's and shoemaker's shops, mortuary and post-mortem room. The nurses slept in rooms on the wards to which they were assigned. There were at first no night nurses, so the staff were effectively on duty almost the whole time. It was envisaged from the start that there might be one nurse per ward, with separate wards for sick and infirm, noisy and refractory, convalescent, and epileptics and paralytics: the last had about a fifth of the accommodation to themselves (see Table 3.2). This is a reminder of what proved to be an important part of the work of the Victorian asylum, the care of the brain-damaged, especially those prone to fits.

The Court of Quarter Sessions approved the architects' plans at Easter 1850 and the building was entrusted to Messrs Holland of Duke St, London, with the iron work of windows and roofs by Cottam and Hillam of Wells St, London. It was ready for occupation by January 1853. Six months before that the Committee had appointed the first medical superintendent, so that he could advise on the furnishing and equipping of the place. Later they appointed a steward and a matron, to organise the asylum to receive its first patients on 17 January. The doctor, John Millar, at first continued in his old job in London, but came regularly to Aylesbury to advise, and he stated his credo in his first annual report:

"everything which tends even in a remote degree to create a feeling of uneasiness or irritation in the mind of the insane is opposed to their successful treatment. . . . I have endeavoured as much as possible in harmony with the building to arrange so that they may not be reminded at every turn they take that they are in a Workhouse or Prison. In their bedrooms, clothing and diet they are better provided than they can be in their own homes, while the domestic appearance of wooden bedsteads, the absence of the badges of pauperism and crime in their dress, the existence of a full diet in accordance with the habits of the middle class and ambition of the poor, leaves them nothing to desire in these essential requisites. . . ."

TABLE 3.2
The size of the female wards in 1853[1]

Nature of ward	No. of single rooms	No. in dormitory	Total
Tranquil and convalescent	8	32	40
Epileptic and paralytic	11	8	19
Noisy and refractory	5	5	10
Sick and infirmary	3	7	10
Chronic	9	12	21

1. The provision for the 100 men was the same.
Note the way the cases were to be divided ('classified').

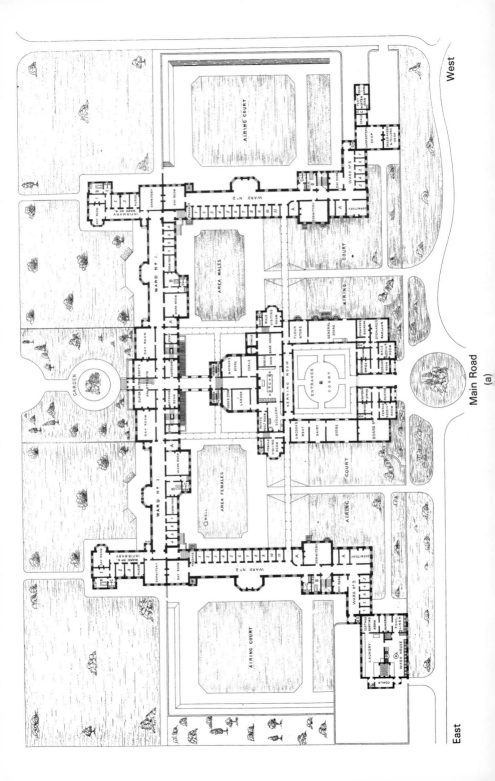

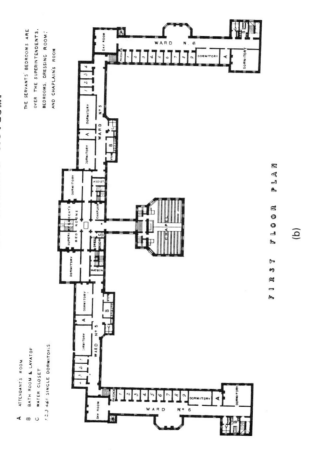

Fig. 3.3. Plans for the asylum: (a) ground floor and (b) first floor. Note that south is to the top of the page

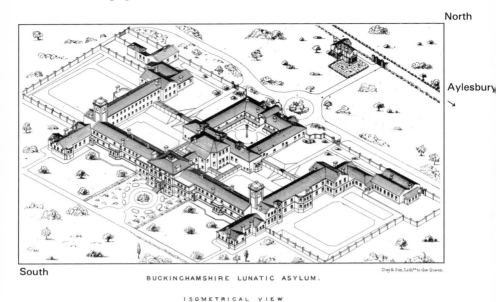

North

Aylesbury

South

BUCKINGHAMSHIRE LUNATIC ASYLUM.

Day & Son, Lith^{rs} to the Queen.

ISOMETRICAL VIEW

Fig. 3.4. A drawing of the asylum as it was to appear in 1853

Horsehair mattresses on canvas spreaders, rugs on the floor and curtains at the windows, bedside chairs, a selection of cotton print dresses for the women and cord suits for the men were other items which later caused the Commissioners in Lunacy to comment on the superior standards offered.

Money

The Committee followed Mr Millar in ordering comfort and amenity in spite of the extra expense. An extra £1490, nearly double the original estimate, was spent on furniture and bedding, the clothing allowance was 50% up, and the slate washing stands and porcelain baths and related fittings, initially costed at £746, became over £1000 more expensive. The original estimate for the land and buildings had totalled £30 500 in 1850, but this had not included separate houses for the engineer and the gardener, the entrance lodge, the stables, farm and garden buildings, or the roads. By 1853 the estimate had risen to £38 500, but when the asylum opened it had cost just over £43 000.

This needed careful justification because there had been opposition to building the asylum all along. In January 1849 about 600 ratepayers, headed by Benjamin Disraeli, had petitioned Quarter Sessions not to proceed, because of the cost (then estimated at £30 000), and the fact that they were already paying for a new gaol and new judges' lodgings. However, the vote had gone 5 to 11 against them, and a loan of £30 000 at 4% interest per annum was negotiated with the Alliance British and Foreign Fire and Life Assurance Company of London (it later had to be increased) against the security of the county rate. This company had already similarly financed the prison.

The first argument the Committee offered was that others were spending similarly. Bucks would have 200 patients at a starting cost of £217 per head; whereas Birmingham, with 312 patients since 1851, had a cost of £238 per head, and Prestwich, with about 400 patients, had spent £193 per head.

The second argument was that an asylum was quite different in function from a workhouse. Its work had a much larger medical component, and it was intended to be a curative institution, not a repressive or frightening or storage one. There was a widely held belief at this time that lunacy was curable if detected in its early stages, and it was hoped that the new asylums would draw in these early cases. The basis for this optimistic view was that some patients did get better after only a short illness (manic–depressives fluctuate between well and ill and well again, sometimes in a matter of only a few weeks) and that in the small private institutions with good care patients often only stayed a short while and were temporarily improved if not cured.

Where the workhouse cost about three shillings per head per week for maintenance, the asylum was nine shillings at Hanwell and eleven shillings at Oxford in 1846, and the cost was to be of this order in the new Bucks asylum.

The cost of care and rehabilitation apart, there was a humane reason for spending more. Mr Millar stated:

> "an opinion which I find in this county [is] that as the insane poor are maintained out of funds raised specially for the support of the Pauper, they are not entitled to anymore consideration nor have any special provision for their care above the condition of persons of the lowest class. . . . Why those suffering from a disorder, the most terrible to which the human race is liable, which the world regards with fear and horror, which affixes a stigma on the sufferer for life . . . should be branded with the vagrant and the mendicant, thus exposed to a degradation . . . which even the committed criminal is spared, appears to me to be an evil which requires amendment. Parochial authorities never complain that convicts cost about 10 shillings a week."

The debate about costs was a long one and still persists. People may be willing to pay for cures, but if the condition is incurable, how much should we spend on chronic disability, what quality of life should be offered? A century later, within the National Health Service, the medical superintendent had to protest because at Christmas dinner the mentally ill at St John's Hospital were allowed a smaller helping of turkey than the physically ill in Stoke Mandeville Hospital; and later, at a time of economy, resisting the administrative suggestion that though the general hospital patients might continue to eat butter, cheaper margarine was good enough for those in the psychiatric hospital.

The willingness of lay people to cut expenditure on the mentally ill arises in part from lack of first-hand personal contact with the different kinds of sufferers, and therefore no feeling for them. They may hold a confused, mistaken idea that the mad have 'lost their senses', that is, no longer taste their food, feel the cold, enjoy bodily comforts; whereas for most patients their discernment and taste are in fact the same as it was before they fell ill. But above all the laymen who control finance have often failed to understand the relation between many diverse items of expenditure and the results they wish to achieve. An asylum or a hospital needs a certain design, a certain staff, a certain medical and psychological technology, if it is to improve or cure, rehabilitate, or simply hold at a given level of individual satisfaction the human beings who come to it. If one or more of the certainties are disregarded in imposed financial cuts, unexpected evils may follow, but the causal link between cut and evil is not always appreciated.

The excessive initial cost of the asylum and the expenses of rectifying the mistakes made over water supply and heating later helped Mr Barker, when he became Chairman of the Committee of Visitors in 1856, to set his face against any further expenditure, even on necessary improvements, and to look to make money by taking in patients from outside Bucks. But in January 1853, when without ceremony the asylum began work, well built and equipped for its time, there was an air of optimism. Its daily life is described in Chapter 7, and some results of care in Chapter 9, but first we shall look at the development of the institution.

Notes

The information in this chapter has been drawn from the early annual reports of the County Pauper Lunatic Asylum (1854 on) and the minute books of the magistrates' committees in the County Record Office. The *Report of the Metropolitan Commissioners in Lunacy to the Lord Chancellor* (1844, London: Bradbury & Evans), but more especially the *Report of the Commissioners in Lunacy to the Lord Chancellor* (1847, London: Shaw & Sons), give descriptions of the best design of asylums and the duties to be undertaken by different members of staff, based on wide inspections of contemporary private and public institutions. An interesting account of the building of a subscription asylum is given by:

FOSS, A. & TRICK, K. (1989) *St Andrew's Hospital, Northampton: The First 150 Years (1838–1988)*. London: Granta.

Additional sources are:

GIROUARD, M. (1979) *The Victorian Country House*. Harvard: Yale University Press.
PEVSNER, N. (1975) *Wiltshire. The Buildings of England* (revised by B. Cherry). Harmondsworth: Penguin.

4 The rise and fall of Mr John Millar

Until the coming of the National Health Service in 1948, the asylums, the mental or psychiatric hospitals of the country, were paid for out of local money and run by local people, without a penny grant from the state. There was of course no Ministry of Health, and other community health provisions were similarly local. The parish doctors appointed by Boards of Guardians under the Poor Law Amendment Act 1834 and the Medical Officers of Health under the Public Health Act 1848 were likewise appointed locally and paid with local money. The only central control of the asylums was vested in the Commissioners in Lunacy (after 1914 renamed the Board of Control), a small London body under the Lord Chancellor. They were led for 40 years by the influential evangelical Lord Shaftesbury, who had made the well-being of the mentally ill his life work. The Commissioners issued detailed instructions on many aspects of asylum work, and sent two of their number for surprise all-day inspection of an asylum once or twice a year. They made criticisms and suggestions, they compared institutions and investigated abuses, and wrote annual reports, but they had very little power. They could try to influence but they could not compel.

The rulers of the asylum were the members of the Committee of Visitors, magistrates until 1890 and county councillors thereafter until 1948. There were usually 14 of them (up to 18 after 1890), including a chairman. It was specified that they were the effective supervisors of the establishment, responsible for all matters of contract and expenditure, for frequent visiting, and for investigating the details of management, the health, physical and mental, of the patients, and the regular keeping of all accounts, certificates and case books. To this end they had to meet every month, and two of them had to visit the asylum and report on it each week. They were appointed annually at Quarter Sessions (or later, by the County Council) and some members served for only one year, although others took a longer interest. Inspection of their minute books shows that often enough in the early days only two or three magistrate members turned up for the monthly meeting, and sometimes it was the Chairman on his own. In consequence the Chairman had most of the power and provided the continuity, controlling above all the money supply. His attitude and his relationship with the chief officers of the asylum were therefore crucial to its success. Table 4.1 lists the Chairmen since 1853.

The Medical Superintendent was the managing director of the institution, the chief adviser to the Committee and responsible for its day-to-day running, which involved instructing and solving problems for the engineer, the gardener, and the lay administrator (steward) and guiding the matron and the chief male nurse and their staffs. This was additional to his medical functions which required seeing all the patients every day, giving all necessary medical and surgical treatment, examining patients admitted on the order of the magistrates, and recommending them for discharge when they were well enough. Note that it was the magistrates, not the doctor, who controlled admission and discharge. However, the morale and the tone of the asylum was set by the Superintendent: if he lost interest the institution decayed.

There had been experiments in two or three places with lay administrators managing asylums, but this had worked badly, and they had been replaced by resident medical officers. Having a doctor full time on site (the Superintendent's house is shown in Fig. 4.1) was better than using a part-time

TABLE 4.1
Chairmen of the Committee[1] 1853–1974, and Medical Superintendents

Chairmen		Superintendents	
Magistrates			
1853–56	George Carrington the Younger	1853–56	John Millar
1856–65	Thomas Raymond Barker	1856–1908	John Humphry
1866–85	Rev. Peter Thomas Ouvry		
1886–89	Henry Bode		
The County Council			
1890–1902	William Lowndes		
1902–3	Edward Terry		
1904–5	Thomas Horwood		
1905–15	Henry Rudolph de Salis	1908–34	Hugh Kerr
1916–27	Thomas Field		
1928–33	Thomas Osborne		J. Shaw Bolton (locum)
1934–48	H. L. Darvill	1935–51	Ian Skottowe
Oxford Regional Board (NHS)			
	L. M. Paterson	1951–61	Samuel L. Last
	K. White	1961–85	David C. Watt (Medical
	C. G. Cousins		Director)
	W. J. Cowley	1985–89	Julian Candy (Chairman
	R. Paterson		of Division of
			Psychiatry and unit
			medical representative)

Oxford Regional Health Authority (after 1974) and District Health Authority

1. As responsibility for the hospital moved from one body to another, there was always a single committee given the task of performing similar management functions.

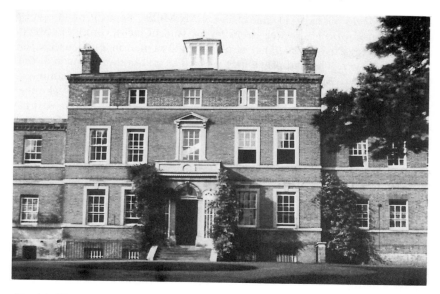

Fig. 4.1. The south front of the asylum: the Superintendent's house

visiting physician or surgeon, and there was a surprising amount of ordinary medical work to be done, quite apart from the belief in the 19th century that madness was a medical problem. It may be also that doctors were generally better educated and had wider sympathies – and were thought more likely to prevent patients suffering from harshness and unnecessary restraint and to encourage visiting by friends – than the exsoldier or the workhouse manager otherwise likely to be in charge.

In June 1852, therefore, in anticipation of the asylum opening in six months, the Committee advertised for a resident medical superintendent, and received 42 applications from doctors. They called a short list of eight for interview, and finally selected Mr John Millar. Then in his late 30s, he had trained at the University of Glasgow (as had three out of five succeeding superintendents) qualifying with the licence of the Royal College of Surgeons of Edinburgh in 1838. As he had no MD he was technically not entitled to be called doctor at this time, and was always addressed as Mr. From 1843 he had worked at a well known private asylum in London at Bethnal Green as a resident assistant surgeon, so he was experienced in the psychiatry of the day. He seems to have been a man of parts. In the course of time he wrote two books, *A plea for the Insane Poor* and *Hints on Insanity*. He became not only a member of the Medical Society of London but a fellow of the Geological and Linnean Societies.

Later in the autumn the Committee appointed as steward and clerk to the asylum Mr Richard Roberts Hollyer, who had had 14 years' experience as a union workhouse governor, the last eight years in Aylesbury. This background was not likely to endear him to Mr Millar, since the philosophies of asylum and workhouse were so different, and in fact a conflict between them soon began to emerge. They also appointed as matron and housekeeper Miss Jane Fryer, who had previously worked as an assistant matron at the Cornwall County Asylum at Bodmin. She was in charge of the female nurses, who were mostly young unmarried women, and was expected to take the chair at meal times in their dining room and act as chaperone, as well as supervise the work in the female wards, which included a good deal of sewing and dressmaking by both patients and staff.

The male nurses, called attendants, were similarly under a chief attendant, and Mr Millar obtained John George from Colney Hatch Asylum for this post. He seems to have had difficulty in recruiting other nursing staff, mostly local people, and the Committee also had difficulty in filling other posts: an advertisement for chaplain brought only one reply, and they decided to ask the vicar of Stone to undertake the work, and he agreed. Mr Hollyer seems to have taken on the cook and domestic staff. The asylum should have opened before the end of 1852, but there was a delay in fitting out the kitchens. The asylum opened on 17 January 1853.

Like a householder in a brand new house, Mr Millar was kept busy from the opening remedying leaking water pipes, smoke and soot blowing down the chimneys in the nurses' private rooms, smelly drains built without traps, fumes from the heating plant entering the wards, and so on. Some of these matters could be put right by the hospital engineer Mr Shrubb, others required plumbers and builders to be called in. The water supply was inadequate, the heating system never seemed to warm the dormitories, and Mr Millar spent time on thermometer readings around the building by night and by day.

On the constructive side the grounds had to be laid out, paved courtyards delimited for the patients to take the air, and gardens planted with fruit trees and bushes. Mr Millar drew up the proposals with the help of the staff, and got Committee approval, for instance, for planting 24 each of pear, plum, damson and cherry trees, 100 each of apple trees, gooseberry, raspberry and currant bushes, and six walnut trees. Equipment was needed: Bibles and hymn books and a harmonium for the chapel, secular books for a library; the nurses wanted to form a band (in January 1855) and the Committee granted £15 for second-hand cornets and horns. They approved the part-time appointments of a singing teacher and a violinist for the patients.

Without secretarial aid, typewriter, or telephone the Superintendent had to do a good deal of writing letters and instructions, scanning catalogues and getting estimates. Fortunately there was a postal delivery and collection every morning, and later the afternoon coach from Thame was arranged to take letters to Aylesbury for posting. There was a good deal of correspondence getting expert advice from heating engineers and learning from other asylums before the heating system could be improved. But lack of water, especially in the summer, presented a major problem. It led at times to cancellation of all baths for patients and to a laundry shortage, and grew worse as the numbers of patients increased.

Measurement of actual water consumption on various occasions showed that the asylum might just get by on 25 gallons per head per day (i.e. for 200 patients 5000 gallons a day). The main well, in an airing court on the female side, only provided 1000–1700 gallons a day, even when the boring was carried to a depth of over 500 feet, and the water was pumped up with a three-horsepower steam engine. The supply proved irregular and died away in a dry summer. An auxiliary well became completely dry. Rainwater off the roof, estimated at 1000 gallons a day, was stored in tanks, and attempts were made to channel surface springs. Water collected from all sources was pumped into four 10 000-gallon cisterns, one in each ventilation tower, one each over kitchen, bakery, and laundry. They seemed to be short by 3000 gallons a day, and needed a three-month reserve supply. Providing storage tanks for 400 000 gallons was not too difficult, but where was the water to come from?

The Superintendent, Mr Millar, and the Reverend J. C. Clutterbuck, a geologist, studied the terrain and decided that across the turnpike road to the north, where there were some sandpits, there was probably a good supply of water in the sand bed which overlay black shale. In 1854/55 the asylum began to pipe water from a sandpit about three-quarters of a mile north-east, paying a rent of £50 p.a. for so doing – but then the owner changed. The Committee tried to buy eight and a half acres round the sandpit from the new owner but the price was too high. Dr Lee, one of their number, offered to sell seven acres of his land further east at Willow Spring for £1000, and to allow access along a private road from the Eythrope road for a nominal sum. This was agreed in 1856. A three-inch pipe was layed to the asylum, and a horse was purchased to drive a pump, which could raise nearly 6000 gallons in six hours. From 1857, then, after four years, the problem seemed to be solved, but at a cost of several thousand pounds.

Today we take an adequate water supply for granted, and it is difficult to realise how hampering it was to rely on capricious wells and springs. On the other hand the Committee hardly responded with any urgency to overcome the difficulties, and were happy to ignore them when preparing to take patients from other counties to make money. Money was always a problem.

By 1871, when the number of patients had doubled, there was again a water shortage, and baths were stopped. Willow Spring seemed to be diminishing, possibly because of low rainfall or because Stone village had grown, with cottagers sinking private wells. They were certainly making new earth closets, and the public analyst shortly warned that Willow Spring water was highly contaminated with sewage and unfit to drink. By this time the Chiltern Hills Spring Water Company had grown sufficiently to be prepared to run a water main to the asylum gate and provide a supply at one shilling per 1000 gallons, say £200–300 a year. However, the Committee preferred to go on trying to modify the works at Willow Spring, and it was not till 1903 that the asylum began to draw partly on the mains supply, and not till 1931 that it began to rely completely on this source for its 30 gallons per head per day.

The patients

To open the asylum, the magistrates agreed the transfer of mentally ill people from the Buckinghamshire workhouses, and also of Bucks-born patients in other county asylums or in private institutions. Thus, on the opening day, 17 January 1853, came 17 residents from the Wycombe Union, and five from Winslow; two days later another 28 patients, and two weeks after that 21 from Peckham House in London, and patients from Wiltshire and Kent. These all had to be examined physically and mentally and their details recorded in the case book, so Mr Millar had plenty of medical work to do. Some of the patients were incurable, advanced in years, and paralytic or epileptic, and some were to die within a month of arrival. Others presented a need for medical or surgical treatment. Thus on 23 April, of six women from the Eton Union, three needed medical care – one had the itch, another ulcerated ankles, a third a purulent vaginal discharge and excoriated thighs. Of the four men transferred with them, one was an epileptic, one too feeble and emaciated to be out of bed, and two were congenital imbeciles.

Some patients who came from home were simply sent to die. One "had been 16 years at home, latterly tied to a chair and [now] perfectly unconscious and reduced to a skeleton"; two "kept at home as long as they could be borne with, one for three and the other for six years, now they are dirty in their habits and too feeble to be out of bed".

They were not all of course like this (see cases in Chapter 1) but a surprisingly large number were. Few of the early supposedly treatable cases came, but unexpected reservoirs of very chronically ill and disabled began to empty into the asylum. This was disappointing to the staff and the Committee, who had hoped to cure in a short time, not care for a long time, but Mr Millar at least held that even the untreatable chronic mental patient ought to be in an asylum where kindness and medical and nursing care were available, rather than abandoned in a harsh workhouse.

He used the annual reports to state his views on such matters, in the hopes of educating his Committee members. In 1853 he writes:

> "I have usually regarded mental disorder, as it is found in asylums to be composed of two great classes: –
>
> 1. Those cases in which the mental disturbance is attributable to moral causes and characterised by incoherence of varying intensity, accompanied by excitement or depression in every degree.

2. Those cases in which with the above state generally paralysis or epilepsy is associated; such as results from injuries, fever, vicious habits etc.; cases of disorder of the senses, idiots and imbeciles.''

He notes that the first group commonly lack sleep and show a loss of weight and a general debility; and therefore tonics to improve digestion, a full and nutritious diet, and sedatives to procure sleep are indicated.

For the second group, the organic brain diseases, there are no curative treatments but nursing care is important. General paralytics cram food into their mouths without reference to its capacity and may choke, unless supervised, with the food chopped small, and moist. Epileptics may bite their tongue or fall and break a bone, or pitch into an open fire during a convulsion, unless guarded at such times. ''With the idiotic and imbecile much may be done by education in correcting the wayward disposition and dirty habits in which they often indulge.''

Note that this is before the days of diagnoses such as manic–depression, schizophrenia, dementia praecox and the like, and that by ''moral causes'' he means psychological, or as some prefer, functional, causes. General paralytics and epileptics, both now treatable or curable, no longer appear in our psychiatric wards, but in the 19th century the two diagnostic categories between them accounted for a substantial number of the 'lunatics' in this Victorian asylum. At this time, too, the mentally handicapped (idiots etc.) had not been separated from the mentally ill. It was not till the 20th century, by and large, that facilities offering the special care they needed began to be planned for and provided.

In his management of his patients Mr Millar followed closely the type of care first developed at the Quaker Retreat in York in the early years of the century, and the non-restraint championed by Conolly at Hanwell from 1839 following its demonstrable effectiveness by Charlesworth and Gardiner Hill at Lincoln. He was proud of the fact that no equipment whatsoever for mechanical restraint existed in his asylum, and that seclusion (a few hours in a padded room under frequent observation) had not been used at all in the first two years of operation. He had tried to provide a home-like environment of a middle-class standard, and claimed the patients responded to kindness and domesticity by not breaking windows or china.

He visited the neighbouring Oxford asylum at Littlemore in August 1853 and came away very critical of many things. Their windows, some covered with wire netting, were so high up the inmates could only see the sky; their plates and mugs were of tin and chamber pots of gutta-percha, there were no separate day rooms for the different sorts of patients, and some of the patients were restrained in strong clothes held by a leather strap with a lock.

In pursuit of his aim of domesticity he allowed his young daughter to go into the female wards with the matron, because it did the women good to see a child, and did no harm to her. He was libertarian, too, in encouraging the patients to leave hospital for short periods, to visit a display of horsemanship, or the Aylesbury fair, or simply to mingle with the citizens in shops and hotels:

> "My own experience and opinion on this question being that the patients selected for such purposes are as little likely to conduct themselves with impropriety as a like number of sane persons in a similar station in life. . . . I consider that the advantages likely to come to the public, from intercourse with the patients, to be far beyond any inconvenience which might follow the practice, because it would tend to remove much of the lamentable ignorance which I find prevails with reference to the actual condition and treatment of the insane."

The members of the Committee of Visitors were at first alarmed at this leave policy, when they became aware of it, and instructed Mr Millar to write to other asylums to find out their practice. Twenty-six superintendents replied, with approval, although warning against allowing patients to visit public houses, and the Committee therefore endorsed the leave policy, with a specific veto, however, on the consumption of alcohol. This was another subject where Millar was libertarian, or perhaps weak. Opposite the asylum on the main road was a pub (it is still there today) where patients working in the asylum's front garden used to go for an occasional pint of beer, quite unofficially. Millar knew this and moved one patient whom he regarded as dangerous away to the other side of the hospital, but as for the rest he said nothing to the landlord of the pub nor to his own staff, and simply noted that the occasional drink did not seem to do the patients any harm.

It was an alcoholic patient who had excited the Committee over easy leave. Charles H was transferred from the Northampton asylum on 1 April 1853 and Mr Millar could detect no mental abnormality in him then or later. He wrote to Dr Nesbitt, the Superintendent of Northampton, and received the reply that Dr Nesbitt had failed to find anything wrong with him either, although he had been admitted with the story that he was violent, and had previously been a patient at St Luke's, in London. Dr Nesbitt had tried to get him discharged, but somehow the Northampton Committee had not been willing. So Mr Millar decided to act, and got his Committee to discharge him home.

Unfortunately, by 13 June he was back in the asylum again, having been drinking very heavily and in a wild state. After nearly three months' sobriety he was discharged home on 6 September, but he was back on 29 October. Again he had been drinking heavily. His wife had thrown him out and said she would never have him back, so he had been taken to the workhouse and there quickly forwarded to the asylum. Again he was a model, sober patient, and in February 1854 asked for his discharge. This was refused, because he had nowhere to live. However, in July the Committee relented and granted it, but now Charles H decided to stay on. On 23 September 1854, he went to Aylesbury on leave in the early afternoon with another patient and Thomas Lissaman, the head attendant, and two male nurses, and only returned at 10.30 p.m., carried back intoxicated and with a head wound received in a fight at the King's Head while the nurses were elsewhere. It was the reverberations of this affair, the details of which were elucidated by the Committee from several witnesses, which led to the ban on alcohol. Nevertheless, a few Sundays later Lissaman was found taking patients into a pub in the neighbouring village of Ford. He was reprimanded and warned, but Millar, as always, tried to defend him, and so attracted adverse comment to himself.

The staff

The Superintendent was at first easy-going with the staff too. When Henry Brown the night nurse came on duty drunk on the night of 8 February 1853, he replaced him by another man for that night, and made Brown pay his substitute's wages for the night, reprimanding but not sacking him. This, said the Chairman of the Committee, would not do: drunkenness should lead to dismissal. Thereafter this rule was applied with some harshness. The shoemaker came back to Stone after an intoxicated evening in Aylesbury, but waited till morning, and sobriety, before re-entering the asylum – but he was sacked. Mrs Clarke, who succeeded Miss Fryer as matron in October 1854 after the latter had resigned, was reported in 1855 by a laundry maid to be drinking spirits, and a nurse who was also her friend came back from leave in London with a hamper found to contain bottles for her. The nurse was at once sacked, and Mrs Clarke forced to resign.

The first chief male attendant, John George, had been dismissed, for reasons not stated, in January 1854, after a year's service, and Millar had written to Lissaman, then at Bethlem, with whom he had worked previously for about five years at Bethnal Green, inviting him to come to Stone. He persuaded the Committee to appoint him, and to increase his salary after a probationary period, and thereafter supported him at all crises, as in the affair of Charles H, and delegated to him responsibilities which he should have kept for himself. From the time of Lissaman's arrival in 1854 there seemed to be a spate of resignations and sackings. Of the seven men and eight women who were nurses in December 1853, only one man remained by the end of 1854. The matron (Miss Fryer) had also left. The reasons for dismissal were given in some cases as "using disrespectful language at the messroom table", "inciting insubordination", "statements injurious to staff comforts and discipline", "ignores matron's and superintendent's suggestions, quarrelsome and dictatorial". Resignations were sometimes provoked by Millar criticising a nurse's work, a reaction which seemed to surprise him, and certainly created difficulty in finding replacements. Some of the new recruits resigned within a month or two of appointment. Three maids and the cook resigned in 1854, and the cook at least returned after Mr Millar's departure in 1856 and gave 12 years' service thereafter.

Mr Millar also found harmony with more senior members of the staff a difficulty. He was annoyed with what he took to be the slow work of the engineer in effecting repairs, and tried to demand detailed dated written statements, which the engineer said he would only give direct to the Committee. He objected to Mr Shrubb having the windows of his cottage cleaned by his assistant, although the windows of the Superintendent's house were cleaned by one of the staff. When Millar forbade Shrubb's children from walking with their nurse along some garden paths on the south of the asylum, the engineer resigned (July 1855).

When Mr Hollyer, the steward, sacked a housemaid for impertinence and inefficiency, Millar shortly after appointed her as a nurse, and when Hollyer protested there was an exchange of intemperate letters and the Committee had to make peace. Millar agreed to withdraw his letter, but said he still felt the same, and that one or the other of them should leave. Extra diets were supposed to be issued to sick patients by the steward in return for a voucher signed by the Superintendent. Millar did not bother to issue vouchers, gave verbal instructions only, then delegated the ordering to the matron and to Lissaman. When it came to a review of the quarter's accounts in April 1856, the consumption of eggs and port appeared to have greatly increased, and the use of soap almost doubled, although the number of resident patients had increased only from 170 to 192 (Table 4.2). Mr Millar was asked to look into the matter, and reported he could see no way of saving on the extra diets, and indeed could propose no changes in general monitoring procedures which might reduce waste or loss. Mr Hollyer on the other hand had suggestions, for example asking matron to keep records of materials used and dresses produced and to return unused material to stores; and making frequent unexpected counts of stores of all kinds. The Committee gladly approved this.

TABLE 4.2
Consumption of soap, eggs and alcohol, 1854–56

Year and quarter	Average no. of patients	Soap: lb	Eggs: no.	Port: glasses	Sherry: glasses
1854					
1	158	932	1038	233	518
2	160	898	1770	463	342
3	165	902	1393	489	69
4	164	818	1839	856	262
1855					
1	169	930	1568	804	273
2	178	1001	2069	944	534
3	193	1083	3265	1428[1]	1063
4	197	1203	3767[1]	1168[1]	897[1]
1856					
1	194	1698[1]	3873[1]	911	814[1]
2	190	1418[1]	3669[1]	769	445
3	189	1353	2435	408	268

1. Particularly striking increases in consumption when the number of patients was constant.

It was at this time that Lissaman was suspected of theft, and stocks of soap, as well as blankets and mattresses from the asylum were found in his house. In conjunction with three other members of staff he was charged and tried before Lord Chief Justice Campbell at the assizes at Aylesbury on 12 July. Two charges were dismissed, but on the third he was sentenced to 18 months' hard labour, and a male nurse, Blackwell, received a six-month sentence on another charge; two other nurses were acquitted. Mr Millar's comment, which did not endear him to the magistrates of the Committee of Visitors, was said to be that robberies were usual in asylums, and could not be prevented. (Indeed, at least twice in later years the chief male nurse was dismissed for dishonesty.)

A whole new area of irregularities came to light when Mrs Bridges came from Slough to claim her husband, an in-patient. Lissaman had ordered Bridges to go to work for Rev. Reade, the hospital chaplain and vicar of Stone, in his garden. When Bridges refused to go he was punished by being put under the cold shower and then locked up, and his wife had heard of this. Although Millar tried to maintain he was not ready for discharge, the Committee decided to hand Bridges over to his wife straight away and he went home, got work, and continued well. Inquiry showed that Lissaman had been sending out patients to neighbouring farms and gardens on his own initiative, without supervision, and had also been using the cold-shower punishment when he wished, although, strictly, only the Superintendent could order such a punishment. Millar maintained he had delegated the use of the shower to Lissaman and to matron: if so he was betraying his patients, because long experience elsewhere had shown that all exercises of power in asylums had to be carefully controlled if brutalities and inhumanities were to be avoided. The Commissioners in Lunacy had a role as official watch-dogs to try to prevent such things.

There was another side, also, brought out by this case. Millar had complained to the Committee that the gardener was too slow in his work, and they had given him notice and advertised for another man. It now appeared likely that he was behind because he had been denied the help of patients, who had instead been sent to help neighbours. Accordingly his notice was rescinded: and he subsequently gave many years of adequate service.

The fall of Mr Millar

Mr Millar had been supported by his Chairman, George Carrington, till at the end of 1855 Mr Carrington resigned on inheriting West Indian estates he had to manage. His work had been approved by the visiting Commissioners in Lunacy, including on three occasions the notable Dr Gaskell, who had made so many major improvements at Lancaster Moor asylum. But now Millar was faced with a new chairman, albeit a man who had been associated with the Committee from the early days of planning, to answer serious criticisms. Matters came to a head at the monthly meeting on 15 August, when there were new allegations that Lissaman had had access to the female side of the hospital and there had been sexual irregularities. The Chairman said they had lost confidence in Mr Millar, and could not go on meeting with him and signing the necessary cheques. He resigned on the spot. A few days later, however, he wrote withdrawing his resignation, and a special meeting was then convened for 29 August at which the Chairman and seven of the 13 Committee members met to consider the crisis. Mr Bernard and Dr Lee proposed postponing any decision till the next monthly meeting but by five votes to three (the Chairman voting) they decided to carry on, and dismiss Mr Millar if he would not resign. He was given three months' notice, and advertisements of the vacancy inserted in the *Times*, the *Lancet* and the *Medical Times*.

This act came as a great shock. Dismissal of a professional man, of an asylum superintendent, was a very rare event, and Mr Millar was determined to fight it. He asked the Committee to specify in writing the precise charges against him, and what exactly Mr Carrington had said in his praise, but they declined to say. He himself listed what he thought were the charges and answered each one, and then circulated a printed pamphlet of denial and self-justification. He appealed to the Association of Medical Officers of Asylums and Hospitals for the Insane (the forerunner of the Royal College of Psychiatrists) and its President, Dr John Hickman, wrote to the Chairman of the Committee asking if he could shed any light on Mr Millar's departure: was he really ignorant of his faults, and would all the facts be given in the annual report to Quarter Sessions? The Chairman replied that they did not recognise any standing of the Association in the matter. Dr Hickman then wrote a second letter, signed by 85 members of the Association, this time to the Lord Lieutenant and magistrates of Buckinghamshire, asking that in common justice the accusations should be made public and Mr Millar allowed to defend himself. This met with no better reply. The Committee said they had full responsibility for running the asylum, and every right to act as they did without wider discussion. Quarter Sessions accepted this; indeed, at their debate it appeared that Mr Millar had no supporters in Bucks (except perhaps Dr Lee). The matter was discussed further by the Committee and by the Quarter Sessions, and no idea of changing the decision emerged. The *Journal of Mental Science*, the Association's journal, in a puzzled comment, opined that Mr Millar's mistake had been not to cultivate the members of his Committee and arouse their interest in the asylum and its work. The written evidence we have (his diary, the annual reports, the Committee minutes) suggests that hasty emotional responses and a lack of judgement, in other words his personality, had also something to do with it.

His fall had such publicity that 25 years later the magistrates of Wells, Somerset, remembered it and asked for details before sacking their own superintendent. Mr Millar himself, after he left at the end of November

1856, took a further medical qualification in 1859 (LRCPEd) and became superintendent back in Bethnal Green, where he continued till his death in 1888.

Notes

It is interesting that other early medical superintendents were dismissed or forced to resign by their committees, notably at Lancaster Moor in 1840 and at St Andrew's, Northampton, in 1845.

The pay of the staff in 1853 is worth noting. Mr Millar received £300 p.a., Mr Hollyer, the steward, £100, Mr Shrubb, the engineer, £90, the gardener £50, the matron £40, and the chief male attendant £35. The stokers got about £33, the lodge-keeper £31, and the male and female nurses £18 and £13 respectively. This was in every case in addition to free board and lodging.

By 1895, partly in recognition of the greater work with so many patients, Mr Humphry was getting £700 and his medical assistant £140, the steward £180 and his assistant £60, the chaplain (non-resident) received £140, the baker £53, the night nurses averaged £36, and the day staff (36 in number) about £25.

When Dr Skottowe came in 1935, his salary was at first £1000 p.a. Like that of the other senior staff it was linked to the number of patients in hospital, and the Bucks Mental Hospital was one of the smaller.

5 Fifty inglorious years

George Carrington of Missenden Abbey had taken a considerable interest in the building of the asylum, and served as first chairman of the Committee of Visitors until he had to resign at the end of 1855. He had throughout been very supportive of Mr Millar, and not overly concerned about money. As a farewell, he donated trees and shrubs for the asylum frontage, and had printed at his own expense an analysis of the problem of adequate water supply to present to all the magistrates. His successor as Chairman, T. R. Barker (Table 5.1), who had also been associated with the asylum from the beginning, was both more conscious of finance and more religious in his outlook: he was an active supporter of Bible societies and of a variety of charities, and also on the Council of the Royal Horticultural Society. It had fallen to him to meet the disturbing revelations of 1856, and to get rid of Mr Millar. Not surprisingly, he and the Committee chose a non-psychiatrist as next Superintendent.

There were 57 candidates for the post, including four psychiatrists who had signed the protest letter from their Association to the Lord Lieutenant. But the chosen man, John Humphry, had never worked in an asylum or private madhouse. He had been for five years resident medical officer in a Birmingham workhouse, responsible medically for over 2000 inmates of whom only 8% were lunatics. While there he had in 1853 taken his licence in midwifery, and previously he had worked for two years in the London Fever Hospital. He had qualified as Member of the Royal College of Surgeons (England) with the Licence of the Society of Apothecaries from University College Hospital, London, in 1849, and was a younger man than Millar. Like him he had no MD and was therefore Mr. He may not have had Millar's specialist knowledge and experience, but he was particularly well thought of as an administrator. In 1855 he had been called to Asiatic Turkey to organise a British civilian hospital in the wake of the Crimean War. Under him the Bucks asylum was to settle into an unadventurous tranquillity. He ruled from November 1856 to January 1908, when he retired aged over 80, and he was to live a further eight years after that.

TABLE 5.1
The Committee of Visitors, with responsibility for management, 1859 and 1891

1859: The magistrates	1891: County councillors
T. R. Barker, Esq., Chairman	William Lowndes, Esq., Chairman
Hon. W. G. Cavendish	Hon. Thomas Fremantle
John Lee Esq., LLD	B. F. Astley, Esq.
T. R. Bernard, Esq.	H. W. Swithinbank, Esq.
G. G. Pigott, Esq.	Mr D. Elliot, butcher
W. Lowndes, Esq.	Mr T. Gurney, gentleman
C. Tower, Esq.	Mr E. Hart, gentleman
P. Wroughton, Esq.	Mr J. F. Pater, farmer
J. T. Senior, Esq.	Rev. G. P. Soames
Rev. C. E. Gray	Mr J. Soper, miller
Rev. P. T. Ouvry	Mr G. Stretton, farmer
Rev. C. Lloyd	Mr W. Taylor, gentleman
Rev. A. P. Cust	Mr E. Terry, farmer
Rev. R. N. Russell	Mr J. Treadwell, farmer

Note that the names are listed in order of social rank, and that W. Lowndes occurs in both committees, while Messrs Barker, Lee, Tower and Senior were members of the original building committee. 'Gentleman' implies simply independent means, whereas an Esquire has an estate.

His first task at takeover was to appoint a new nursing staff. The old staff had been sacked, or resigned with Millar, and there were about 15 vacancies. He advertised and had 42 applicants; among others he took on both John Batho and his wife, from Southwark, and after two weeks promoted him to head attendant. Meanwhile the existing matron, Maria Nicholls, was twice in trouble – once when Mrs Batho reported that the equipment of her ward was deficient by the inventory; and again when women patients were found to have their hair badly infested with lice. She had nothing to say on either matter. She was given notice, and a Mrs Caroline Thompson ruled in her place, only to be sacked in her turn. Mr Humphry then appointed Mrs Helen Aitken, matron of the Epping Union Workhouse. With Mr Hollyer, that made three of them workhouse-trained. Two of the new male attendants soon complained to the Committee in writing that the chaplain had been interfering in their work and off-duty time. The Committee did not hesitate to reprimand the Rev. Reade for this, although he was a gentleman like the magistrates themselves, and not a commoner like Mr Humphry. (The Post Office Directory for 1864 listed all the inhabitants of Stone in two groups: first the gentlemen, like the Rev. Reade and Dr Lee of Hartwell; then separately the commoners.) A year later, when he became vicar of Ellesborough a few miles away, Reade resigned and the Rev. Charles Lowndes of Hartwell took over.

One or two people who had resigned because of Mr Millar now returned. Humphry also made use of an agency, the Metropolitan Servants Institution (1857) to gather a new team round him.

His second task on arrival was to inspect his asylum. He reported that it could easily take an extra 80 patients, who could come from outside the county and therefore be charged, to yield a profit. Of course, the asylum had been carefully designed for 200, but this could be ignored by a man with experience only of workhouse standards, and the Chairman was keen to go into business. Few private patients could be expected, but groups of patients could be accepted from other county asylums and charged at a profitable rate.

The transfer of groups of disabled chronic in-patients for months or even years was a common practice between 1850 and 1949. An asylum which was having considerable building operations, or was temporarily overloaded, or which (in wartime) was taken over as a military hospital, could move its residents elsewhere for an agreed fee. The recipient asylum could use its spare capacity (when it had any) to make money, to the benefit of the local ratepayers. The possibility that such transfers might be inhumane, like eviction from one's home away from familiar friends and neighbours, was not considered, although some transferred patients complained to the inspectors. It is true that those selected for transfer tended to be the idiots, the quiet demented, the speechless – those most disabled and presumed to be least sentient. The recipient asylum could regard them as incurable and neglect them, far from their relations, who might have forgotten them anyway. The basic objection to these block transfers was that it treated human beings like things, and this is an attitude to be fought at all times. It easily spreads in institutions, with a consequent growth of neglect or active cruelty.

A glance at the journal which the Superintendent had to keep and show to the monthly meetings of the Committee gives an idea of his day-to-day work. Here are some excerpts from 1858.

4 January "W Jerome readmitted after an absence of 3 years. Mary Bushnell admitted as a private patient, being the subject of suicidal melancholia and in feeble health."

11 January "Mary Palmer age 36 died 5.30 am of general paralysis. I have today suspended Isabella Stevenson from performing her duties as Night Nurse, for absenting herself from the asylum last night and all today, not only without permission but after I had expressly forbidden her doing so. (Discharged)"

12 January "J G Beesley admitted, the subject of acute mania and in ill health."

13 January "R Haddenam age 33 died 3.30 am of cancer of the brain. Mary Bushnell age 56 died 2 pm of pneumonia, having been in the asylum 9 days."

18 January "Sarah Palethorpe commenced duty as night nurse. She has good testimonials from the Lincoln asylum, where she lived 4 years. J G Beesley age 38 died 9.30 pm of exhaustion from acute mania."

23 January "Sarah Palethorpe does not like the duties of night nurse and wishes to leave as soon as her successor can be obtained."

4 February "G Swindon age 21 died 2.30 pm of epilepsy."

11 February "Sarah Palethorpe left today and Catherine Hamilton succeeded her."

24 February "I beg to recommend to your notice as fit for discharge J East and H Butcher and to request that an allowance of 10s be made to each of them. I am also of the opinion that Lucy Smith has recovered sufficiently to warrant her discharge on probation, with an allowance of 3s 6d per week for 3 weeks.

Number in the asylum	92 men	119 women
employed in some way	48	73
attended chapel	59	52
sick	5	5 ,,

5 March "I visited the whole of the patients between 10 and 12 pm: all were quiet and comfortable."

9 March "J Williams admitted in a state of furious excitement. He was bound hand and foot by ropes."

24 March [The Committee asks about prayers.] "They are now attentively read by an attendant in each gallery while the patients are seated at table after breakfast and supper, and thus all hear them, whereas when I read them daily in chapel last year not more than one third of the men and one fourth of the women attended."

21 July "An extra male attendant being much wanted in the men's refractory ward . . . I have temporarily engaged J Richmond aged 22, shoemaker of Haddenham, at the usual wage of £20 a year, and he entered on his duties today.

30 July "Six male patients transferred from Notts Asylum." [A further five men were transferred on 6 August, and 5 on 23 August, or 16 in all.]

1 August. "H Plested age 43 admitted in great excitement, and with a fracture of the Right Leg." [He was fit for discharge on 19 November.]

15 November "By permitting the patients in No 6 gallery to dine in the recess, I have been enabled to place 10 beds in the room lately used as a dining room, and thus to increase beds on the women's side from 130 to 140."

20 November "Mary Ann Smith (a patient in No 8) last evening secreted a pair of scissors and early this morning wounded herself in the throat. Fortunately she only cut a large vein, and though much blood has been lost there is no immediate danger."

1 December "H Cooper age 80 admitted as a private patient."

10 December "Mr Cooper removed at my request as I did not consider it necessary for him to be detained in the asylum."

16 December "Attended board meeting of the Commissioners in Lunacy in London: Mr Cooper's case thoroughly investigated."

23 December "I have summarily dismissed attendant H Luce for returning drunk after two hours' leave of absence in the middle of yesterday."

What is typical here of the entries is the amount of physical illness and the number of deaths – including a death from manic excitement, which today no longer happens. There are also sidelights on the recruitment and discipline of staff. Alcoholic intoxications continued as a staff problem. John Batho was sacked in May 1860 for stealing asylum property (and was imprisoned for nine months) and another chief attendant likewise in 1864, confirming Mr Millar's tactless remark of 1856 about asylum robberies. However, the next man stayed 11 years, until his retirement through ill-health.

In the report of their annual inspection on 29 November 1861, the Commissioners in Lunacy found all the patients well clothed and their personal state very satisfactory. All the wards were remarkably clean and cheerful:

> "The various dormitories and single sleeping rooms are provided generally with bedside carpets, with chairs, with muslin blinds and with curtains of white dimity; the beds are all of horsehair and the bedding excellent. . . . Entertainments, comprising music and dancing, at which the patients of both sexes associate, are now given weekly and about 100 generally take part. . . . We saw the patients at Dinner. It was neatly and well-served and consisted of meat and vegetables, both very good and supplied in abundance. . . . [The patients] appear to be treated with great kindness by the nurses and attendants."

The Bucks patients, incidentally, were costing 9s or 9s 6d per week, and others were charged at 1s 9d extra – a profit.

Epilepsy

Mr Humphry only once used his annual report to educate the Committee, and that was at the end of 1861 when he gave an analysis of the amount of epilepsy in the hospital, no doubt because it gave the nurses a great deal of work and was an argument for increasing the staff. He said the number of epileptics was slowly increasing, in spite of some deaths (three in the year). There had been 5766 fits in the year. One man alone had had 1183; but the other 42 epileptic patients (16% of the patients) had averaged about ten fits a month each, and many of these attacks required nursing care to prevent self-injury. Some of the fits were followed by periods of violent behaviour, which also needed handling, including sometimes a period of seclusion of the patient. The difficulty of the nursing care of epileptics became more noticeable when such patients died in the night from an unobserved fit in which, turning in bed while unconscious, they suffocated themselves.

Coroners' inquests on such cases were reported in 1866, 1871, and 1872 (two cases in the year), and led the Commissioners in Lunacy to demand that something be done to stop this loss of life. Visiting once an hour at night, Mr Humphry's first response, was no good, and putting the most at risk of the epileptics and suicidal in a 12-bed dormitory with a night nurse did not answer either. After more fruitless advice, in 1875 the Commissioners said he must do what other asylums did, bring all the epileptics together (males and females separately, of course) and have a nurse sitting up all night with them, to spot the fit at once. The Committee responded by sanctioning the employment of two more night nurses, and one by day, and since there were no dormitories big enough to hold the 25 epileptic men and 29 epileptic women then resident, they agreed to building operations on two ground-floor dormitories to double their size and add four side-rooms to each, giving space for 34 of each sex. When all the epileptics had been brought together, the problem at night was solved, but not until two more patients had suffocated themselves, and the two nurses who had failed to watch them sufficiently, contrary to the new rules, had been sacked.

Now another difficulty was reported by the inspecting Commissioners: not enough day space for the epileptics. They had been brought together from different wards for the night, and to send them back every day to the places whence they came was very unsatisfactory.

The Committee under Mr Barker was very unwilling to embark on any big expenditures, and procrastinated, and Mr Humphry does not appear to have been a man to challenge them on behalf of his patients. The solution to the epileptic deaths was delayed several years. The Commissioners had meanwhile also been commenting recurrently on the insufficiency of the infirmary wards, in their reports of 1868–76 and onwards without any notice whatsoever being taken.

It is true that the building and repairs account (supported by the county rate, plus any profits made from patients from outside Bucks) shows an annual expenditure from about £900 to £1800. Occasionally the Committee might be tempted into a bigger expenditure. One of the earliest was the very necessary enlargement and modernising of the laundry in 1862, which became a steam laundry at a cost of about £400. It was able to undertake much more work, but more economically, with a saving on soap, and an easing of unpleasant work for the patients.

When the pressure on space kept on mounting with more and more patients, Mr Barker relented somewhat and called in Mr Brandon, the architect, to add 50 beds for women. Mr Giles Holland of Thame submitted the lowest tender (£2406) and built the extension, but they made him pay 10s per day for his water from the asylum. With delays the extra beds were ready about mid-1865, when on grounds of infirmity and age Mr Barker resigned from the Committee.

From the start of 1866, therefore, there was a new Chairman, Rev. Peter Thomas Ouvry, a member of the Committee since 1858. He was to hold office for nearly 20 years. He was in general more responsive to the suggestions of the Commissioners in Lunacy than his predecessor had been, and less rigid in his financial prudence, though continuing the policy of trying to make a profit out of some patients.

Fire precautions

The Reverend Ouvry and the Committee were quite prepared (in 1877) to beautify the asylum with a splendid (public) turret clock (Fig. 5.1) mounted

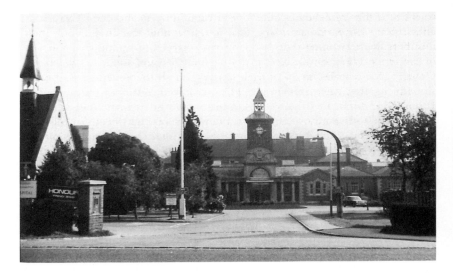

Fig. 5.1. The entrance from the main road on the north. Note the turret clock of 1877 and the new chapel of 1869 on the left

in a tower with weather-vane and lightning conductor, at a cost of £525. They were slower however when it came to fire precautions, and here Mr Humphry appears to have been partly at fault since there were no planned exits in case of fire, nor even any official instructions what to do if a fire broke out.

When the Commissioners discovered this in 1877 they were astonished. The Committee took the view, however, that their building having been constructed with fireproof iron window frames and iron ceilings and concrete floors, there was little risk. When the Commissioners continued to be critical in 1878 they bought "three small engines, such as are usually used in watering gardens . . . besides three hand pumps intended to be used in a pail of water". The discovery of this by the inspectors brought a polite but fierce letter from the head office in Whitehall asking the Committee to look at the matter of fire quickly and seriously. In January 1883 the Commissioners noted the existence of a fire-engine in its shed, but regretted that no fire brigade had yet been organised, nor rules drawn up. This was six years since the matter had been first mooted, hardly a rapid response to an important safety measure. Now exits in case of fire were marked out for the patients, and later some iron escape staircases added. At last a group of male staff started fire-training under the new resident engineer, Mr Edwin Field.

Setting up the brigade aggravated an old and ever-growing problem of how to house the staff. Mr Humphry had been at his wits' end to find how to squeeze in more and more resident nurses, and at least once had failed to fill a post established by the Committee because there was no room, although the Commissioners were frequently commenting on the inadequate numbers of staff. Married men had been allowed to sleep out, but the men of the fire brigade obviously needed to sleep on or close to the premises. Cottages for married men on the land just north across the road seemed the answer, and some other asylums had already found this a good idea. Proposed in 1884, three pairs of cottages were ready a year later at a total cost of £1200 – the management could move fast enough when it wanted to.

So finally, by 1886, there were fire rules, exits and an asylum fire brigade. Unfortunately, or fortunately, it had nothing to do. When the inspectors rang the fire alarm on 19 April 1898 a manual fire-engine "of antiquated pattern" worked by 16 patients under four nurses made its appearance and it was nearly half an hour before water could be laid on to the building.

During 1904 periodical fire drills began, and all hydrants, hoses and appliances were overhauled and supplemented. This was just in time for the brigade's great moment. At 9 a.m. on 9 January 1905 fire was discovered in the roof of the nurses' quarters in the new building (open less than one year). By the time the Aylesbury Town Fire Brigade arrived things were largely under control. Damage was assessed at £301–5-10d, and the Alliance Insurance office promptly paid up. Fire-proofing was adopted in the rebuilding.

In the printed *General Rules for the Government of the Bucks County Asylum* (1914) we find on p. 31 "Rules for the Engineer and Clerk of the Works as Chief of the Fire Brigade" specifying a weekly test of fire-alarm bells throughout the asylum, testing all hoses to withstand pressure twice a year, protecting with straw all outside hydrants from freezing in winter, keeping records of all drills, tests, practices and the names of those involved, and instructing all staff in use of extinguishers and rescue of patients. So at long last proper fire precautions were in operation.

Swelling numbers

Asylums had been opened with the promise that they would offer cure, but the reality proved very different. Year after year in his annual reports the Superintendent was to write such sentences as "of the 421 lunatics resident at the end of the year only 18 can be considered curable, and probably several of these may not realise the hope of recovery now entertained" (1869); "Of the admissions during the year a proportion amounting to nearly 40 per cent were from the first seen to be hopelessly incurable, and of the remaining cases in many instances there is but little chance of their recovery" (1876).

To understand what was happening let us look at a few figures from 1861. The asylum took in 79 new patients in the year and discharged as recovered or improved no less than 32 (ten years later, in 1871 the figures were 78 and 51), so total pessimism was wrong. But the trouble lay in the nature of some of the cases. Old people past work and with their relatives dead are more likely to stay in hospital whatever their illnesses, and in both 1861 and 1871 17 patients aged over 60 were admitted, or roughly a quarter of all admittances. It is true that some of these people died within the year, 5 in 1861 and 13 in 1871, but the more usual thing was to survive.

Another growing group was the mentally handicapped, the imbeciles and idiots from birth, who once admitted were likely to stay, and certainly could not be expected to grow in intelligence. Some of them were epileptic. Table 5.2 gives figures for 1861 and Table 9.3, p. 120, compares the figures every tenth year to 1911 and shows how these categories of incurable increased and helped to choke the asylum.

Pressure also came from another direction. The February 1863 county return of 'known lunatics' showed 232 in the asylum, plus 57 in Buckinghamshire workhouses, plus 84 at home or with friends. As the

TABLE 5.2
The asylum's work in 1861

	Patient numbers
Admissions	
In asylum on 22 December 1860	243
Admitted	79
Discharged	34 (23 recovered, 9 improved, 2 unchanged)
Died	18
Escaped	1
Transferred elsewhere	3
Total in asylum on 31 December 1861	266
Nature of patients admitted	
(a) Diagnoses	
epilepsy	8 (total of 43 in asylum)
severe mental handicap	4
general paralysis of the insane	2
partial paralysis	2
melancholia	15
excitement	39
other	9
(b) Aged over 60 years	17
(c) Origins	
Bucks 'paupers'	63
private patients	8
Oxford contract	7
Surrey contract	1
(d) Chronicity	
new cases	50
second attack	16
third attack	7
fourth or more	6

Note that 34 discharged as against 79 admitted is a discharge rate of 43%, and that patients could be discharged and then readmitted in later years, and discharged again.
Note also the importance of epilepsy and old age – 21.5% of admissions were aged over 60.

century went on there was a growing tendency to move patients from home, or from the workhouse, to the asylum: there is a particular comment on this in the 1911 annual report, a year which saw 47 patients over 60 and 22 mentally handicapped as well as 12 with general paresis (due to syphilitic infection of the brain) form 42% of the total admissions from Bucks in that year.

Back in 1866 Mr Humphry had summarised the situation for the Committee. It was already a national tendency, not a Bucks idiosyncrasy, this rapid asylum expansion with incurables, and it gave rise to anxious discussions whether the whole nation was going mad, degenerating perhaps through some ill effect of civilisation or industrialisation. No one knew whether there was a real increase in the amount of mental illness or not and certainly the number of chronically disabled people in the community had been very underestimated. Better food and sanitation were prolonging people's lives in or out of hospital; the criteria for admission to hospital had perhaps softened, and public attitudes played a part in this; and certainly more complete and accurate statistics were being recorded. So the 200 beds of the asylum of 1853 were bound to be inadequate sooner or later, though this was something the Committee reluctantly discovered by degrees as the years went by.

Profit making

The Committee compounded the inadequacy by repeatedly trying to make money from extra patients, either private or under contract made with some other county. In 1884 an analysis of the patients of the three preceding decades was performed (Table 5.3). On average in the first and third of these decades a quarter of the asylum population was admitted to yield money, and yet it did not in the end yield very much. In the first decade, when the asylum cost about £8000 per annum to run, there was an average annual profit of about £127; in the third, when the running cost was about £13 000, the profit had risen to about £600 p.a. or 4½% on cost – they were then charging 14s extra per private patient per week, as opposed to 1s 9d at the beginning. But these profits were actually less than appeared because the resultant overcrowding of the asylum brought various extra expenses, of which having to expand the buildings sooner than would otherwise have occurred was one. However, as the profit was credited to the repairs account funded annually by the county, it made a difference of 10–30% to the total available sum, which was not inconsiderable.

Mr Barker, who introduced the profit-making policy, tried to set his face against any expensive new building when the asylum had been so expensive to create initially. The inspecting Commissioners in Lunacy were quick to comment on the overcrowding. It was not just a matter of the single rooms having two beds squeezed in, or the dining rooms being turned into additional dormitories, or even that two lavatories were not enough for

TABLE 5.3
Free and profit-yielding patients

	Totals admitted in 10-year periods		
	1853–62	1863–72	1873–82
Number of Bucks 'paupers'	744	741	821
Number of private patients	40	41	72
Criminals (court orders)	5	15	9
Contract and out-of-county cases	155	61	162
Ten-year profit on non-Bucks cases	£1276	£3444	£5958

50 patients, or three wash-basins for 40 men, but that the laundry (and later the kitchens) were too small to cope with the extra work, and a new, bigger chapel was needed if 160 of the patients were to attend religious services. In the end he grudgingly permitted the new enlarged steam laundry of 1862 and, as already recorded, allowed the building of an extra 50 beds for women (since the overcrowding was worse on the female side) in 1865 as he retired.

First expansion

The new Chairman, the Rev. Ouvry, was more willing to allow expansion. Mr Brandon was called in to add accommodation for 50 more men and 50 more women, and to design a new and separate chapel to hold 240; so that the old chapel, after strengthening the floor, could become a recreation hall (Fig. 5.2). Quarter Sessions approved the plans, and the estimated cost

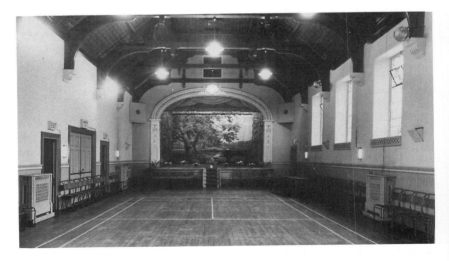

Fig. 5.2. Interior of the original chapel converted to a recreation hall (taken in 1962). Dances, badminton, drama and cinema shows were held here

including finishings and heating plant was £10 000, in July 1867. The work was offered to Mr Robert Ellis Roberts of Islington at £6429 for the main building and £1713 for the chapel. By December 1868 the ground floor on the male side was already occupied, and the women were about to enter their new ward, but the new chapel could only be opened in June 1869, because of a difficulty in getting facing stone from a local quarry.

The Commissioners had emphasised the need for more land – the original 20 acres (for 200 patients) plus the addition of a seven-acre field nearby was now quite inadequate (for almost 400) – but finding it was not easy. Inquiries met with refusal from the vicar of Stone and from a farmer on the west, but suddenly in 1869, owing to another farmer's death, there was the possibility of buying 26 acres just across the road from the asylum, at a cost not exceeding £3000. The Court of Quarter Sessions agreed to this, and the land became asylum property on Lady Day 1870. Although it was intended in the first instance to provide opportunity to the male patients for farm work, it came opportunely for the provision of a burial ground. Stone villagers had complained through the vestry that their church graveyard was becoming full of asylum dead, and the Commissioners in Lunacy agreeing after discussion, an area was surrounded by a stone wall and consecrated by the Lord Bishop of Oxford on 2 August 1871 and used almost at once.

During 1868 the average number of patients in the asylum had been 342; during 1869 it rose to 398. The Committee recognised that one doctor by himself could not reasonably cope with so many, as the Commissioners had been pointing out for some time. They decided the matron was unnecessary, and her work could be undertaken by the existing senior female attendant. This saved a salary of £50, and a flat, and thereby they could now house an assistant medical officer. Dr W. Bevan Lewis, MRCS, LRCP, trained at Guy's Hospital London, was appointed from 1 March 1869 at a salary of £80 p.a. Very much later he was to become a very prominent psychiatrist.

The growth of the asylum had led to Mr Hollyer, the clerk and steward, getting an assistant in late 1866. In 1875 Mr Hollyer began to be ill, and eventually unable to carry on his work. He resigned in January 1876 and died three days later. During all the time he was off sick, and during the interruption until the new man Mr W. H. Sharman was appointed and took over, Mr Humphry carried out the duties of clerk and steward as well as his own. The Committee was so impressed with this display of administrative capacity that they made him a gift of £60.

The number of nurses also was increased in stages, but since they had all to be resident it began to be difficult to find them accommodation, and some of the single rooms intended for patients began to be used. They also received pay rises, notably in 1873. By this time there were 20 nurses and 14 male attendants, plus two night attendants on each wing, more than double the numbers when Mr Humphry had started 17 years earlier.

One of the first results of the new wards was to relieve the overcrowding, but the Committee at once took on 70 patients from London workhouses: 60 were chronic mentally ill or defective but 10 were thought potentially curable. It meant money again, and it filled the free space more or less, only the Committee and the Commissioners in Lunacy disagreed as to how big this space was, by about 40 beds. These contracts for out-of-county patients were always for a maximum of five years at a time and could be shorter if necessary, although the Committee was loathe to do this.

Quality of care

Overcrowding was liable to spread tuberculosis and dysentery in the asylum, though this was perhaps not appreciated at the time. Overcrowding certainly made the assessment of the patients less efficient, and made it more likely that recovery would be overlooked, at least for a time, and consequently discharge unnecessarily delayed. The case of George Channer is probably to be explained in this way. He had been accused of housebreaking in 1881, aged 23, found insane, and sent to the asylum. In January 1885 Humphry reported to the Home Office that he was fully recovered and fit for discharge. In the following ten months he continued well, but Humphry heard nothing from London and did not write again. When the Commissioners inspected in October they discovered this, took the matter up, and Channer was released at once, and subsequently did very well.

The Commissioners repeatedly criticised the lack of nurses, and they used various objective measures to show the insufficiency of care. The number of patients wetting the bed at night was one. If every patient is got up regularly to urinate on a three- or four-hourly basis, there should be no wet beds at all. The number with bedsores was another. If bedridden patients are turned frequently in bed they should not develop bedsores. The Commissioners were very insistent that all patients who died should receive a post-mortem examination, because this would lead to reports of terminal bedsores or unexpected causes of death (choking on food for example) indicating lack of care. Post-mortems also of course were a check on the doctor's care in examination and diagnosis.

In the 1860s and '70s, while critical of the drains, the accommodation, and particular matters such as fire precautions, the annual inspectors usually ended with praise for the general running of the asylum. From 1876, however, they began to complain that only a third of the deaths were followed by a post-mortem examination; and it was not till 1889 and the years thereafter that post-mortems were performed for two-thirds of deaths and more, rising to over 90% in 1897. At the same time they began to comment on the number of the dead found to have bedsores at post-mortem – 13 out of 36 in 1895 and 10 out of 42 the following year. As for wet beds, these were anything from 20 to 40 on the night before they visited in the years from 1888, when they began a renewed onslaught on the overcrowding. Once again, single rooms had two patients, dormitories were overflowing, yet there were claimed to be 46 vacancies – the Committee repeatedly claimed the asylum held 480 when just full, and the Commissioners responded that on the basis of floor space and the evidence of their eyes 420 was the upper limit.

Second expansion

On 26 April 1889 the newly set up Buckinghamshire County Council took over from the magistrates in Quarter Sessions the control and finance of the asylum, while the Lunacy (Consolidation) Act 1890 changed the rules for dealing with the mad. The change in management meant a completely new committee (except for one member) and a big one, from around 12 up to 18 members, and a new Chairman, William Lowndes, who as a magistrate had been a Committee member at the start, 36 years earlier. Instead of magistrates appointed by the Lord Lieutenant, there were to be councillors elected by democratic vote. The number of country gentlemen and Anglican clergy decreased, and businessmen, shopkeepers and farmers began to take their place (Table 5.1). This in itself meant a more careful financial policy, but also a lessening of direct financial understanding. Henceforth the Visiting Committee of the asylum was to be subject to the remote Treasurer and Finance Committee of the County Council, instead of to brother magistrates in Quarter Sessions, but their management role continued as before.

There was almost immediately a big change. For years the maintenance charge for Bucks 'paupers' had been of the order of 9s or 9s 6d. Now the asylum Committee cut it to 7s or so, chiefly by reducing the food and stopping the allowance of beer patients had hitherto always enjoyed. Thereafter in annual report after annual report they showed a weekly maintenance cost always about 1s cheaper than the average cost per week in the asylums of the whole country. From time to time the annual inspectors commented on the serving of a meagre dinner of watery soup and bread, or rhubarb tart and water as the only course of the main meal.

At first the new Committee, unlike the old, used to answer the Commissioners back, point by point, asserting the diet was adequate, or those who needed more could have it, or (more generally) that everything possible was being done. Perhaps this was chiefly to satisfy the County Council, or to create an appearance of rugged independence from London. In fact, the answering back died after a few years, and while yet still offering anodyne answers or protests in their reports, they began in practice to adopt some of the Commissioners' suggestions. Cheese was added to a meal of bread and tea alone. They resumed making helping gifts of money to some patients discharged from the asylum on probation (which the old Committee had granted without question) when the Commissioners commented that most asylums found it a good idea.

The public attitude to the mad had hardened. They had become frightening and must be locked away. They would probably never come out again, unless they escaped, because there was no cure. The Act of 1890 was to safeguard the citizen from being wrongfully incarcerated, and make sure the lunatic was neutralised. There was, too, something reprehensible about being a pauper, a suspicion still that madness arose from moral weakness and sin. With these attitudes it becomes comprehensible why the county councillors, grudging money spent on food, entertainment, and nursing (which they did not understand anyway), were yet quite agreeable to put up big new buildings to enclose yet more lunatics. They had responded to the Commissioners' suggestions by building bedrooms and a common-room for nine nurses (opened 1891), and providing more day space for women, at a cost of almost £1100, and then, in 1895, spending £540 on improved sanitary annexes, with pedestal toilets. New workshops costing £740 were opened in February 1899.

Meanwhile, the overcrowding had become such that the Committee had regretfully to send back all contract patients and forego the profit, and resolved to have a new building to hold an additional 200 patients. Mr R. J. Thomas, County Surveyor and architect, prepared two alternative schemes, one a separate building across the road on land to the north, the other an extension of the existing buildings, which the Committee favoured. The Commissioners in Luncy would only approve this, however, if at the same time they bought more land. They managed to acquire 20 acres on the west for £2250. While this was going forward, they made a contract with Hertfordshire County Asylum at Hill End, St Albans, to take 20 women patients for up to three years, at £780-15-0 for a full year.

Messrs W. Pattison of Rustington, Sleaford, were appointed to put up the building. They were permitted to take for their offices rooms occupied normally by night nurses, who had to be squeezed in elsewhere; and the laundry was closed and the work was instead sent to Aylesbury launderers for the time being. It was decided to take the opportunity to supply the asylum with electricity throughout. When the building, at a cost of £59 102, was opened 29 February 1904 (Fig. 5.3), it had wards for 113 patients of each sex, an enlarged chapel and recreation hall, a water main linking 18 fire hydrants, increased kitchen and administrative space, and quarters (''Eskdale'') for an assistant medical officer and 21 nurses. With all this the burial ground was enlarged and consecrated by the Bishop on 20 January 1905. The new organ for the chapel was paid for by a legacy from Mrs Ann R. Jarvis, willed in 1877 and invested since. She had wanted to do something for the patients.

Thus the asylum had been enlarged to take about 620 patients (about 700 in the Committee's belief) and they promptly made a further contract for 60 London patients at 14s per head per week.

Now, having passed his 50th year as Superintendent, and been ill twice, Mr Humphry decided in January 1908 to retire, and Dr Hugh Kerr, his

North

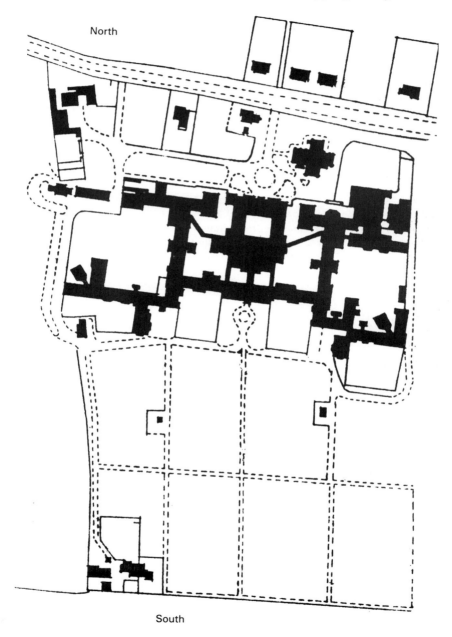

South

Fig. 5.3. Plan of the hospital after the second expansion, of 1904. Note the three pairs of cottages for nurses, built in 1885, on the land purchased in 1870 north of the main road. The new chapel is just south of this, and the gas-works with engineer's and gardener's cottages are at the south-west (bottom left) corner

assistant medical officer, was appointed to succeed him. Humphry had seen himself always as the servant of the Committee, not its guide and teacher, and in no sense an innovator. All the changes involved in the growth of the asylum had been pressed on him by the Commissioners in Lunacy, even in quite minor matters, and he seems to have had little imagination, and no marked concern for his patients, at least in the last 20 years of his long rule. Neither he nor the Bucks asylum was in any way noteworthy in the English asylum world, and this at a period when British psychiatry generally had sunk into an impoverished routine, while the progress was being made in Europe, particularly in the Germanic university clinics.

Notes

The information in this section is drawn from the asylum's annual reports and the Superintendent's diary.

6 Cold storage

Hugh Kerr, who became Superintendent in 1908 and so continued till his death in 1934, was about 40 years younger than Mr Humphry, and better educated. After graduating with an MA in 1887 he took the medical course at the University of Glasgow, qualifying with commendation in 1892 and winning the Mackintosh Prize in mental science. He had then worked in the county asylum at Abergavenny for four years, before coming as assistant to Mr Humphry in 1896. He continued studying while working, obtaining his MD at Glasgow in 1899, the same year in which he published articles on recurrent insanity, and on congenital malformations of the ear. In 1904 and 1905 he had papers in the *Lancet* on "Spontaneous rupture of the heart in an insane patient" and "Mental symptoms associated with heart disease", but published nothing more once he was Superintendent.

Soon after his arrival he was put in charge of nurse training. Since 1891 the Medico-Psychological Association of Great Britain and Ireland (the fore-runner of the Royal College of Psychiatrists of today) had held examinations for a certificate "in nursing and attendance on insane persons", and provided from 1885 the first textbook of nursing. From 1898 Dr Kerr had prepared his students for this examination and was able to boast in 1910 that 50 of them had passed, and that 21 of these certificated nurses were still on the asylum staff. The Committee kindly granted them an extra £2 a year in recognition of the certificate.

Under Humphry in his latter days nursing care had frequently been criticised at the annual inspections. Kerr, perhaps because of his closer contact with the trained staff, was able to see a reduction in the number of beds wet at night and in the number of patients with bedsores; in fact 1910, 1913 and 1914 were years in which not a single bedsore was reported. The annual reports also show the decline in the number of fractures each year, more likely to be suffered by elderly and feeble patients when there is insufficient nursing care and overcrowding.

Kerr had nearly seven years of peace until World War I. This was a time when he not only improved the nursing and softened the Spartan rigours of the diet somewhat, but promoted a plan of regular redecoration of the wards and introduction of minor physical improvements. The building was getting on for 60 years old in its greater part, and antiquated in design compared with the new asylums of the 20th century. It needed doing up and refurnishing. His annual reports are much more informative than Humphry's and show at first some interest in epidemiology and inheritance of mental illness.

In his second report (in 1909) he included a table showing how the number of known 'insane' in Bucks had increased between 1895 and 1905 out of all proportion to the population growth at the end of the 19th century. A greater number of patients were coming into the asylum, instead of staying at home or in the workhouses. He noted particularly a rise in the number of the senile (over 65 years old), who previously would not have been certified, and in the numbers of idiots and imbeciles. Thus, resident in the asylum in 1890 were 52 imbeciles and 17 seniles, compared with 97 imbeciles and 29 seniles in 1910. In 1910 there were in all 622 patients, so the old and mentally handicapped formed a fifth of the total.

The congenitally mentally handicapped worried the Commissioners in Lunacy because it was by then recognised that they needed different treatment from the mentally ill. The Idiots Act 1886 had already distinguished the handicapped, like that from infancy and failing normal mental development, from the ill, normal people who had been struck in adult life by a mental breakdown. The Commissioners were particularly worried by the mentally handicapped aged under 15 (in 1910 nine boys and five girls) who they thought ought not to mix all the time with adults, and ought to be getting some education. But the Committee and Dr Kerr took no action of any kind, presumably not regarding it as their concern. At that time there were a few beds in the Winslow and Aylesbury workhouses for the mentally handicapped, but otherwise the asylum was the only place they could be sent. Buckinghamshire County Council took a long time to be pressed into providing for them: 16 years later they opened Manor House in Aylesbury, and seven years after that (1933) joined with other authorities in opening Borocourt Hospital near Reading.

It is true that the Lunacy (Consolidation) Act 1890 had ignored the distinction made in the 1886 Act and defined "a lunatic as an idiot or a person of unsound mind". This may have been responsible for the increase in admission of imbeciles noted by Dr Kerr. But it is also possible that thanks to better public health, more imbeciles were surviving into later childhood. It may also represent a development of public opinion towards the segregation of the abnormal which the Lunacy Act as a whole expressed.

The 1890 Act, which lasted till big changes in 1930, compelled the County Council to maintain the asylum, and to appoint from the councillors the Committee of Visitors which inspected the institution every month or more often, appointed the senior staff and controlled all finance, and made the policy. The Superintendent was their employee but alone held the legal responsibilities of the institution. He had to see that only patients duly certified, and correctly so, were admitted; he was responsible for holding them and seeing they were treated as the law layed down; he in the first instance controlled their discharge. Because of this he was required to be resident at all times, unless a deputy could be found. Because of his legal responsibilities he might, one would have thought, have been able to frighten the Committee into providing more help and more facilities by saying that otherwise he could not properly do his legal duty. But Dr Kerr never seems to have attempted this in his earlier years and from 1916 was faced with a strong Chairman, with his own ideas.

The 1890 Act provided that, as before, it was a magistrate who ordered a patient into the asylum, and the asylum to take him, but the reception order had to be accompanied by evidence from a doctor or doctors of his mental abnormality (the certificate). Any doctor and any magistrate were sufficient for this, supported by a policeman, relieving officer, or overseer of the poor. In other words the asylum doctor, with knowledge and experience of mental illness, took no part in identifying a lunatic, and had no possibility of refusing to take anyone sent in, even if the asylum was full. This was a recipe for overcrowding, of course, though after the new building of 1904 the asylum was not full again till about 1912. The asylum doctor was not required by law to treat or to discharge the patient again, but of course if his special knowledge allowed it, so much the better. What he did have to do was keep numerous record books of the patients so that inspectors could check on what was going on, and in particular he had to be responsible for humane care. This meant a daily or twice-daily perambulation through all the wards, and a look behind any locked door to make sure no patient was imprisoned. Seclusion was not permitted to the nursing staff – only the Superintendent could order it, if he thought fit, the order being given in writing in a special book, indicating for how many hours it was to be allowed. The patient was to be inspected every half-hour and reported in writing, and to be let out again at the end of the ordered period, unless a new order was written. The inspectors were always very interested to know how many patients were being secluded, for how long, and why, and this helped to keep the amount of seclusion down.

From 1908 to 1912 Dr Kerr had as his assistant Dr J. F. Carson, who then joined the Colonial Medical Service abroad. His successor Dr F. D. Crossthwaite stayed nine months and then went to South Africa. A rapid turnover of medical assistants meant that they might know little and be of less use. The care of 600 patients was a big task, and needed more than one assistant. The Commissioners on their annual inspections kept on urging that a second assistant be appointed. It was not till 20 years after the start of World War I that such a thing came to pass, forced by peculiar circumstances.

The small size of asylum staffs and the long reigns of superintendents made career prospects poor in the mental hospital service and encouraged leavers.

Apart from medical and surgical care for the physical health of the patients, regular reassessment of their mental states, guarding their humane treatment, post-mortem examinations of all the dead, training the staff, watching over the kitchens, the laundry, the engineer's department, the buildings and the estate, the Superintendent had to cope also with new official requirements. Following the passing of the Factories and Workshops Act 1907, factory inspectors began to call regularly and point out dangers which needed correction. Fencing and guarding was needed in the laundry, where a woman patient crushed her fingers. The pumping engine for the water supply had to be fenced in in 1911, and so on. The Asylum Officers Superannuation Act 1909 meant calculations of wages and benefits in the various occupations to determine the proper monthly or weekly contribution to the future pension. In 1911 the Committee raised the wages of nurses and artisans to cover the cost to them of their weekly contributions, and gave married men who lived out an extra lodging allowance in place of board and residence.

Pay and terms of service were beginning to matter more, as the mental hospital world became more professional and distinct. A National Asylum Workers Union was founded in 1910, one of the roots of COHSE, the Confederation of Health Service Employees of today. The employers' side met in the Mental Hospitals Association, formed in 1918 just in time to negotiate with the union in 1919 on nurses' hours of work and wages. Mr Field, Chairman of the Bucks Asylum Committee from 1916, was a prime mover in founding this association, and became its first treasurer. He was supported actively in this by several members of his Visiting Committee.

The distinctness of this world was shown by the appointment of new staff always from within it. When in 1913 Miss Millard, the chief female nurse, retired on pension after 25 years' service, Miss Baird from the Prestwich asylum (Manchester) came in her place; and when she moved a year later to be matron of Brislington House, a noted private asylum near Bristol, she was succeeded by Mrs Haythornthwaite from the Wiltshire county asylum. In 1914 Mr A. T. Hobley, the clerk and steward, retired through ill health, and was replaced by Mr E. J. Jeffries, chosen from 66 candidates, previously an assistant at Essex county asylum, at Colchester. Mr Edwin Field, the engineer who had been promoted clerk of the works (and chief of the fire brigade) retired in 1915 after 32 years' service, and Mr B. J. Baker from Graylingwell asylum (Chichester) was chosen from 104 candidates to follow him.

So the Edwardian years of peace quietly ran out. The pumps for the deep well were renewed, the 25-year-old cooking equipment in the kitchens overhauled, and 27 acres of the vicar's glebe land purchased for £2000 to use for sewage disposal. The hospital heating system had grown to depend on 17 separate boilers and instead of piecemeal renewal from time to time the Committee planned one central system.

Meanwhile the old problem of overcrowding came up once again. The Commissioners pointed out in 1911 and again in 1912 that there were too many women patients for the space available – and in 1912 there was an outbreak of dysentery among them, 25 cases with one death, to drive the point home. Further building was required, and in 1913 they recommended giving some thought to the asylum's special requirements. If a new nurses' home was built, nurses would no longer have to occupy single rooms on the wards, which could consequently house additional patients (and the nurses would much prefer this, aiding recruitment of additional staff). If open-air verandahs were provided for the nursing of the tuberculous in accord with modern ideas of treatment, the spread of the disease might be controlled. If a separate admissions ward or unit was built for the new patients, they could be kept apart from the chronically disturbed, the mad and the epileptic, and the senile, making it easier (and less upsetting to them) to treat them.

The Committee accepted the need for new buildings and began drawing preliminary plans. Meanwhile, they followed up two other suggestions for reducing overcrowding, by discharging harmless chronic long-stay patients who could do without asylum care. One plan was to invite families to take their certified relatives back – but there were no takers. (No doubt financial cost to the family fuelled their unwillingness.) The other plan was to invite workhouses to take these harmless chronic patients. Most refused, although one or two gave it a try, but the patients so transferred were back in the asylum in a few months. Building plans went on. The outbreak of war, August 1914, put a stop on all such building projects – as far as the Bucks County Council were concerned, because some projects did continue up to 1916 in other areas as the annual reports of the Board of Control indicate (in 1914 the Board replaced the Commissioners in Lunacy, little more than a change of name).

The disaster of 1914–18

The War Office needed military hospitals to treat large numbers of wounded, and with the agreement of the Board of Control they took over a number of county asylums, and other asylums had to accept and house their displaced patients for the duration of the war, at basic cost. So in March 1915 Bucks received 29 men and 35 women from the Norfolk asylum, and a further 33 men and 38 women from Northampton in November. Since Bucks asylum was full before any of these transfers arrived, the overcrowding produced was on a scale never before seen. Extra beds were squeezed into the dormitories, the corridors filled with beds, other rooms were converted into bedrooms. This was a body blow to the asylum.

A second blow was the departure of over half the total strength of male nurses for the Forces – from a staff already judged too small by the annual inspectors. By the end of 1915, 16 men had gone. Seven labourers (mostly from the hospital farm), a painter, a bricklayer, a stoker, a tailor, a carpenter and a baker had also been lost. The men were not replaced by women, as happened in some other asylums. Women were said to be unobtainable, but perhaps there was also a local feeling against women nursing mentally abnormal men. By July 1918 the male nursing staff was only 17 strong (with four night attendants and seven charge nurses). The female staff were 24 with five night staff and eight sisters. The roll of honour in 1918 showed 34 male nurses and 22 artisans away on active military service, with eight killed in action. Figure 6.1 shows Dr Kerr with 23 male nurses in 1920.

It is not surprising if, with this staff deficit, and the increase in numbers of patients (including an extra 30 from Littlemore in 1918, and 46 acute admissions from Oxon and Northants) the nursing became minimal, and the death rate soared. It is also noticeable that the number of patients of both sexes discharged as recovered or improved fell to about half its usual annual size – either recovery was impaired, or the recovered were never noticed in the crush. The one bright spot was that the admission rate for men was noticeably down throughout the war – that for women was also reduced for the first two years – otherwise the overcrowding would have been even greater.

A third body blow was the Committee's determination to keep down running costs, at a time of rising prices. They twice in the war years had to raise the pay of the staff to match the rise in the cost of living – this was general throughout the country. But they could save on the patients' food (see Chapters 8 and 9 for details). There was no official food rationing till 1918, but they cut the patients' rations to keep the weekly maintenance from rising as fast as it would otherwise. It was 9s 4d per week in 1914, rose to 10s 6d in the latter half of 1915, to 11s in 1916, to 12s and about

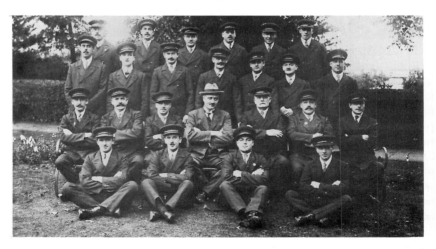

Fig. 6.1. The Superintendent, Dr Kerr (centre), with 23 male nurses in their uniforms, 1920

13s in 1917, to over 15s by the end of 1918, and quickly soared to 25s in 1919 as the food policy of the hospital became more generous, after the staggering death rate in 1918.

The result of the food cuts was a progressive rise in deaths in each year of the war. The deaths were about 67 for each of the five years 1910–14, rose to 81 in 1915, 110 in 1916, 129 in 1917, and 257 in 1918. Most of these deaths in 1918 occurred before the arrival of the great influenza pandemic in the late autumn: only 22 patients died out of 291 cases of influenza (7.5%, compared with three deaths out of 51 cases among the staff, 5.9%). In each year, too, the death rate from tuberculosis shot up. When one considers that the total patient population was less than 800, it appears that in 1918 about one-third of all of them died: it certainly relieved the overcrowding.

All the Committee had to say, in their 1916 and 1917 reports, was "the general health of the patients has on the whole been satisfactory". Dr Kerr in his report for 1917 wrote:

> "the increase in the death rate amongst the older and more feeble patients and the increase of tubercolosis must be attributed in part to the altered conditions, and indicate that a generous diet is necessary for the maintenance of the vitality of the insane."

So gently put, this was hardly likely to penetrate the hearts and minds of the Committee. In any case the deaths rose at all ages and not just among the elderly and feeble (see Chapter 9).

In fact many asylums showed rising death rates during the war, though Bucks was almost the highest of all. The Board of Control became perturbed, but unwilling to explain it, because the rise varied from place to place and was not shown by all. Many superintendents, however, gave it as their opinion that lack of enough food was an important cause. The Board ended with a metaphorical shrug of the shoulders: after all, everyone had to make sacrifices for the war effort. The 300 extra dead at the asylum have no war memorial, but they too were casualties of war.

Soldiers and sailors discharged from the Services as insane were admitted to county asylums as a new category of "service patients" who would not carry the stigma of being paupers. They were to be treated as private patients, paid for by the Ministry of Pensions, and with a special visiting service. There were never very many of them at the Buckingham County Asylum – a peak of 50, but more often 20–30. Many stayed a long while – some were still there 40 and more years later. This may have played a part in softening the general public attitude to mental illness. There had been a lurking suspicion that people brought madness on themselves, through intemperance for instance. However, it was easy to believe that our brave boys had been driven mad through no fault of their own but by the hell of war in the Flanders mud and therefore to become more sympathetic.

The war brought three minor but significant changes to the asylum year. The annual reports stopped publishing statistics of the history and progress of the patients in care – initially to save the labour of compiling them and the paper they were printed on, but when peace came the figures and tables were not resumed. This betokened a certain loss of interest in the therapeutic and diagnostic work of the hospital. It was becoming more of a storage warehouse. Likewise the chaplain's annual report was dropped after 1915, and never resumed. Alongside the official (Anglican) chaplain there were now a Roman Catholic priest and a Nonconformist minister who also did ward visiting and were allowed an occasional service in the chapel, but who wrote no reports. In fact the importance of religion in the life and treatment of the hospital had shrunk and would shrink further to a minority position all round (see also Chapter 8).

The third change was that, understandably, the land used for recreation by the patients in peacetime had been ploughed up to grow food during the war. But now the war was over it did not revert to its recreational use but became an experimental farm, as discussed below. This was again a sign of a certain lack of interest in and concern for the patients.

A businessman's hospital

The war ended in November 1918 at the height of the influenza pandemic, and when in addition to all the staff laid low by it, Dr T. S. Logan, assistant medical officer through all the war years, died of it, the hospital was paralysed for a time. But then Dr Mark Anthony was appointed (he was to serve till Dr Kerr's death in 1934) and 24 male staff returned from the war, and things looked up. At the Board of Control's suggestion Dr Kerr was now weighing patients every quarter: with improved food rations they were no longer losing weight and many were beginning to gain a little. The era of semistarvation was over, and the annual death and discharge rates reverted to their pre-war levels.

Mr Rudolph de Salis had been Chairman of the Committee for 11 years till the end of 1915 when he resigned, though remaining a Committee member for a while. The new Chairman, Alderman Thomas Field, had an optician's shop in Aylesbury, and lived with an unmarried sister; in 1916 he was in his early 60s. He was an altogether more enterprising force. In 1918 he called a meeting at the Guildhall in London as a result of which the Mental Hospitals Association was founded. He took with him in support such Committee members as the Mayor of Aylesbury, and Alderman Thomas Osborne, a mayor of Buckingham who became Chairman of the Bucks Mental Hospital Committee after Mr Field's death in 1928. They took part in early discussions with the Board of Control to establish the new category of voluntary (informal) patients which they favoured; and they were advocates of economy in hospital administration.

The name was changed from Bucks County Asylum to Bucks Mental Hospital, and Mr Field, foreseeing a growing demand for places for private (profit-yielding) patients, ordered the preparation of two wards (100 beds) ready to receive them. This plan was foiled by a sudden official request that they should house 74 Littlemore patients for two years while Littlemore continued as a Ministry of Pensions neurological centre; and by an increase in admissions from Bucks itself. The likelihood of overcrowding, and the plans of 1913 and 1914 for extra buildings, seemed quite forgotten. The plan for centralising the hot water and heating system was resuscitated however, and in 1920 two large Lancashire boilers and a 500-gallon calorifier were installed.

Mr Field prudently managed to build up the repairs and maintenance fund (which he could use without involving the County Council Finance Committee in pleas for money) till it reached £29 000 in 1923, and drew heavy criticism from the District Auditor. In the following years, therefore, it was used to reduce the weekly charges per patient exacted from the parish unions, so that by 1927 the balance was only £19 000. It would have been better from the patients' point of view if the money had been used to improve the sanitation and the care of the tuberculous, both very poor and repeatedly criticised, but it was not.

Money was not lacking for other physical improvements, however. In 1922 a cold-storage plant was installed for £515, and electric cooking and baking equipment for £800 plus a new dough mixer for £396. The scale of the new kitchen equipment was quite interesting. Two 20-gallon stock pots and four roasting ovens, plus an 80-egg boiler, a fish range with steel canopy, a grill and four hot cupboards are listed, as well as two baking ovens to cook 1000 lb of bread in six hours. The electricity needed for this new equipment was supplied by the hospital's own power station. The electric kitchens and the power house were shown with pride to a group of mental hospital engineers from London and elsewhere who visited in September 1925; a photograph of the main control and distribution switchboard for the kitchens had been published a few months before in the hospital's annual report, curiously the only photograph ever to appear in the reports.

The hospital farm as an experimental station

What stands out as one of Mr Field's special contributions to the mental hospital was his promotion of the hospital farm. It had expanded during the war by taking over land intended for the patients' recreation, and now a seven-year lease of 32 acres of Upton Farm (at £80 per acre) was added, a new poultry house built, and a one-acre fruit orchard created. This was all in co-operation with the County's Agricultural Instruction Sub-committee, begun in 1922. Various experiments were tried, as summarised in the hospital's annual reports: spring manuring of wheat, variations in pig feed, production of winter eggs, trial fruit growing, effects of various manures on potatoes, mangolds, swedes, and clover. Seeds and artificial manures were supplied free of cost to the hospital Estate and Farm Sub-committee, the hospital's employees did the work, and the crops could be used by the hospital either for sale, or to supplement the patients' diet.

The scale of the work can be illustrated by a few figures. In 1925 there were 324 hens plus 206 pullets and 188 cockerels; over 50 000 eggs were laid in the year, 10% of them in the autumn quarter when eggs were dearest. In 1930 this had increased to 500 laying hens and 385 ducks. With the help of a motor tractor and plough purchased in 1927 there were in 1930 15½ acres under wheat and another 31½ acres ploughed; in that year too there were a boar and seven sows and 62 store pigs. The farm in 1930 represented rather more than 10% of the annual running cost of the hospital as a whole (£4569 against £44 430). Provisions for patients and staff cost £12 409, but of this the farm contributed £535 as eggs and poultry, £872 as potatoes and vegetables and £522 as pork. Farm wages were estimated at £1475, and purchase of provender etc. £594, so the food benefit to the hospital in terms of cost was nil. The figures can be compared with other costs such as printing, stationery, entertainments, etc., at £1493, or £252 spent on medicines and surgery.

The original point of the farm back in 1860 had been at least partly to provide occupation for male patients who came from a predominantly rural county, but the towns in Bucks had grown, so fewer men were agricultural labourers. The farm had been improved to yield either useful practical results from experiments or profit from the sale of its produce, which meant that only productive, hard workers were wanted – patients working for nothing. Not many patients were suitable by the 1920s, no more than 38 out of a total of 260 in 1929, while another 22 worked in the workshops, three in the bakehouse, and eight in the stores. This left 169 men unoccupied (though a few may have helped with the domestic work in their wards). Of the 357 women there were 32 in the laundry, 12 in the kitchens and 110 said to be sewing, leaving 203 unoccupied except for possible domestic work. Some patients worked well and saved the hospital employing waged staff. Others did rather little, but received benefit socially. Sometimes the nurse supposed to look after them did more farm work or sewing than nursing.

Hospital care stagnating

The inspectors from the Board of Control frequently criticised the lack of occupation for many of the patients. The hospital lacked suitable variety, it lacked space, and it lacked staff with the time to promote it. The Royal Commission report of 1926 spoke approvingly of occupational therapy, and proposed there should be a staff member in each hospital to specialise in patient employment, in and out of hospital. Work was seen as stimulating, providing interest in place of boredom and apathy, giving a framework to the day and the week, improving social contacts which patients needed. As a result of action by two women members of the Committee in 1932, a six-month experiment was finally begun in which a visiting instructress in handicrafts would teach selected patients. Mrs York came from Eton (at £4 per week including travelling expenses) and started with about 20 patients. Her initial reports, and those from the staff, were encouraging, but she resigned at the end of the experiment, when the Chairman thanked her and opined that nurses could carry on the work now she had shown them how. The problem of occupation had to wait another 20 years before it began to be solved.

The importance of social aid to patients was also not grasped by the Chairman nor, presumably, by Dr Kerr. Most asylums gave at least some financial aid to patients on discharge from hospital, and under the magistrates this had happened in Bucks too. But the County Council dropped the practice, and later reintroduced it for a few selected patients only, in spite of comments from the Board of Control suggesting it might prevent readmission. In 1923 Mrs Broadbent, the first woman on the Committee, circulated a printed address by Dr J. R. Lord, an eminent London psychiatrist and editor of the *Journal of Mental Science* on "Social workers and the insane". This made the points that wise counselling might sometimes avert an attack of mental illness; that admission to hospital might leave a family without its breadwinner, or without the mother to care for children, or could put the home at the mercy of neighbours or a rapacious landlord; and that people often needed help after discharge from hospital, to re-establish themselves. Since 1879 there had been in London a voluntary society, the After-Care Association, to help expatients. It had been founded on the initiative of the chaplain of Colney Hatch Asylum at Friern Barnet in north London. But every hospital needed such a service. Mrs Broadbent's initiative led to some discussion, and finally sank without trace when the Committee issued a general appeal for voluntary lady visitors. That was the last heard of social workers until 20 years on. The first professional full-time appointment came in September 1945.

Dr Kerr was in his 50s when the war ended, and seemed to have lost enterprise and initiative. He does not seem to have been able to stand up to Mr Field, or to fight for any improvement for the patients, or even for himself in getting more medical assistance. His work deteriorated to such an extent that the Board of Control inspectors on their annual visit in March 1932 wrote some biting things about him. They asked if he was aware that Iuminal (phenobarbitone, discovered in 1912) had proved very successful in preventing epileptic fits, and if so why did he not treat his patients with it? Examining the records of three patients who had recently died from general paralysis of the insane, they saw that none of them had been offered the malarial treatment (discovered to be effective in 1917, available in the London area from 1926 or before), and why was this? The 14 deaths from tuberculosis were too many: why were there no facilities for its early diagnosis, such as examination of sputum for the presence of the causative bacilli? They asked again for the provision of a small laboratory for routine tests such as this, and for open verandahs where those with active tuberculosis could be nursed apart from the others and so be less likely to infect them. Since 1916 each patients had had a separate case paper or chart (before that they were all written in turn into the same book), but even these medical records were being poorly kept. The Mental Treatment Act 1930 had provided that patients could be admitted without certification as voluntary (i.e. informal) patients. In Bucks, however, most patients were still certified (only 11 voluntary admissions in 1931 and 19 in 1932). The Act had also provided for the setting up of out-patient clinics, and Dr Kerr had been glad to let others provide in his county. The Institute of Medical Psychology provided one in the south, in Windsor, the Radcliffe Infirmary at Oxford would suffice for the centre, and Northampton General Hospital for the north. In fact Dr Kerr and Dr Anthony, his assistant, had already far too much to do to be able to do it properly, let alone change and expand, but they were clamped into a rigid hierarchical unimaginative routine.

However, one small valuable innovation did occur. In 1923 Mr Field agreed to regular visits by a dental surgeon, and allowed patients to have eye tests and spectacles without charge from his own firm in Aylesbury. He also, with his sister, generously presented the first ''portable wireless installation'' and a silent cinema projector for the benefit of the patients at a special ceremony attended by Sir Frederick Willis, KBE, CB, Chairman of the Board of Control, and other distinguished guests. Figure 6.2 shows a cinema programme of the time, and Fig. 6.3 a drama programme.

When Field died in May 1928 he was succeeded by Alderman Thomas Osborne, a man of the same stamp who had been on the Committee since 1916. He began to change some of the policies, until, aged 74, he was forced to retire after only six years.

Thus in 1930 the hospital decided to get all its water supply, 25 000 gallons a day, from the Chiltern Hills Spring Water Company, under a ten-year contract initially. It was the year in which it bought its first motor transport, a one-ton Morris commercial van for £220. In 1932 it bought a talking film projector – compelled to it, since it was becoming impossible to hire silent films to entertain the patients.

The year 1931 was one of slump, stock-market crash, national financial crisis, and devaluation of the pound. In common with other bodies, the Committee took the occasion to cut wages and salaries as their contribution to financial recovery. Farm workers and tradesmen continued without cuts at their negotiated pay rates, but the rest of the staff lost 2.5% where they earned up to £200 p.a., then 3.75% on the next £100, 5% off the next £250, and so on. It lasted only for the year of 1933 and then the cuts were restored.

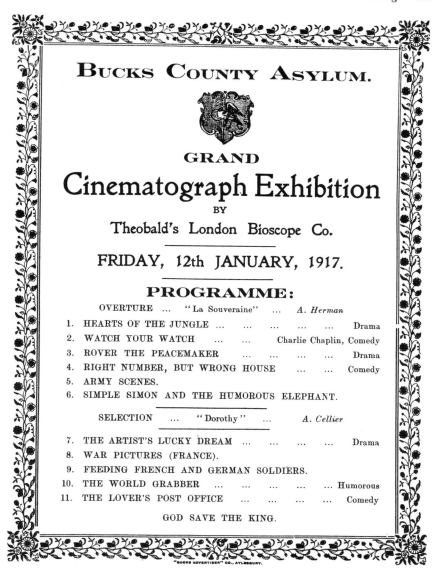

Fig. 6.2. A silent film programme from 1917. Note that the hospital orchestra played two pieces as well as accompanying the films

The biggest change over which Mr Osborne presided was the attitude to further building. Since 1925 the Board of Control had been pressing for more accommodation because of overcrowding and Mr Field had responded annually with a series of excuses – they must wait for the Royal Commission

BUCKS MENTAL HOSPITAL.

WEDNESDAY, 31st DECEMBER, 1924.

New Year's Eve Entertainment.

" The Purse-Strings "

A COMEDY IN FOUR ACTS.   By BERNARD PARRY.

Characters :

EDWARD ASHBY, K.C.	Mr. E. J. Jefferies.
JAMES WILLMORE	Mr. R. W. Ward.
MR. BEAUCHAMP (A Solicitor)	Mr. H. H. Noble.
MARY WILLMORE (Willmore's Wife)	Mrs. Kerr.
IDA BENTLEY (A Widow)	Mrs. Jefferies.
SUSAN (A Servant)	Miss M. Sexton.

ACT I.
Scene—Garden at Willmore's house, Walton-on-Thames.
Time—A Morning in May.

ACT II.
Scene—Morning Room at Willmore's house. Six weeks have elapsed.

ACT III.
Scene—The same. A month later.

ACT IV.
Scene—The same. Five months later.

OVERTURE .... "Raymond" .... Thomas
THE ORCHESTRA.

Music between the Acts.

Violin—Mr. J. W. VERITY.   Piano—Mr. BEVAN MAY.

(a) " Mélodie" .... Rubinstein
(b) "Le Rêve" ....─...................... Goltermann

" GOD SAVE THE KING."

BUCKS ADVERTISER CO., AYLESBURY.

Fig. 6.3. A drama programme from 1924. Mrs Kerr, the Superintendent's wife, played leading parts and sometimes produced; Mr Verity, chief male nurse, played solo violin and conducted the orchestra; Mr Jeffries was hospital secretary and Mr Ward was his assistant

report in 1926, they must see what pressure on the workhouses to take chronic patients would do (failed before, and of course failed again), they needed more land and no one was disposed to sell, the vicar of Stone was ill and could not negotiate, and, finally, that until the cost of the 1904 extension was paid off (sometime in the '30s) the Committee could not envisage spending on a new building. Under Mr Osborne the Committee changed its mind and conceded new buildings were needed. They began to consider drawing up plans, and developing them in detail, under continued pressure from London. By 1931 the inspectors were pointing out that there were 50 more women than the sleeping spaces allowed, there were only two toilets for 60 women in Ward 10, and that most wards had no running water.

In fact the Committee was forced for the first time in very many years to board out patients in other hospitals – and pay for them. It began with 19 women sent to Bodmin in Cornwall for three years in 1932, and then 20 women and up to 20 men at Littlemore.

By January 1934 they at last managed to purchase 21 ⅔ acres of the Stone vicarage estate, including a cottage and the vicarage itself, for £4000, also a 13-acre field (Great Howards) for £350, and the 32 acres of Upton farm they previously had rented, for £900. They developed plans for a 60-bed separate admission hospital, three separate villas of 50 beds each, a nurses' home for 40, and a new house for the Medical Superintendent so that his old quarters could house a third doctor.

When Mr Osborne retired in March 1934, Mr H. L. Darvill took over as Chairman. He was 70, a chartered accountant and director of the Slough and Eton Building Society and the Slough Gas and Coke Co., and a justice of the peace. He had been only a few months in office, when suddenly in November 1934 Dr Kerr died (there has been a memorial tablet to him in the chapel since 1938), and all plans were suspended until a new superintendent could take office and approve. In the ordinary way Dr Mark Anthony could hope to succeed, but he fell ill in January 1935.

This precipitated a real crisis. With no doctor at all the hospital could no longer function, legally, medically, administratively. By a stroke of good fortune Professor Shaw Bolton, a former director of the West Riding (Wakefield) Mental Hospital, had just retired from the Chair of Psychiatry at Leeds to live at Beaconsfield in Bucks. He was willing to act as a locum resident superintendent, provided there were *two* experienced medical officers to help him; and Dr S. R. Tattersall and his wife Dr Edith Booth arrived from Lancashire to do so. Professor Bolton was known as a vigorous independent administrator, who had often acted on his own initiative first and then invited his Committee to approve, which with grumbling they usually did – quite a contrast to Mr Humphry and Dr Kerr. He was well placed to advise the Committee how backward their hospital was, and to encourage them to accept the suggestion from the Board of Control that a special advisory committee with expert knowledge should help in choosing the new Superintendent. This idea had originated with the Royal Commission in 1926. Out of 39 applicants, Dr J. S. Ian Skottowe, then aged 33 and already Superintendent of Cefn Coed Hospital at Swansea, was chosen. Like Dr Kerr and Mr Millar before him he was a Glasgow graduate (MB, ChB, 1923; MD with commendation, 1930). He had been a Henderson research scholar in mental diseases, and then assistant physician at the Boston (USA) Psychopathic Hospital linked with Harvard University. He had published a number of papers – "Management of psychoses of middle life" (*Lancet*, 1929), "Diagnosis of psychoses of young adults" (1930), and "Utility of psychiatric outpatient clinics" (1931) in the *Journal of Mental Science* – and was altogether more original and more experienced than his predecessors.

Thus 1935 was a turning-point, a new beginning. There was a new Chairman, new medical staff and new Superintendent, and outside adviser (Dr Shaw Bolton remained as honorary physician till his death).

Back in 1924 William Crouch, a solicitor who was clerk to the Committee, had resigned after 35 years' service, to be succeeded by his son, Guy Crouch, who continued till the start of the National Health Service in 1948. Dr Kerr had been 38 years at the hospital, and Mr Humphry over 50. Clearly the atmosphere had been one of long service, but that too was now to change.

Notes

For biographical information see *Who's Who in Bucks* (1936), and Dr Shaw Bolton's obituary in the *Lancet* (November 1946). The County Council's annual diary also provided information for this chapter. The medico-social history of Friern Hospital (Colney Hatch Asylum) shows many similarities with that of the Bucks County Asylum, with both good and evil in common – see:

HUNTER, R. & MACALPINE, I. (1974) *Psychiatry for the Poor*. London: Dawson.

III. Eighty years of nursing

7 Love, discipline and money

The asylum, the mental hospital, St John's, aimed to offer protection, board and lodging, and something more: treatment. Treatment was only to a minor extent surgery or medicine because there were almost no physical treatments of mental illness until after 1918, and really effective medicine for some mental illnesses only came after 1953 (see Table 9.2, p. 119). Of course the physical health of the patients required care, and there was more ill-health about than in a general-practice population of the same size, partly because of the greater proportion of elderly in the asylum. But in any close community infections easily spread (Florence Nightingale wrote papers about the death rates in Army barracks due to poor hygiene). Also, some patients, from the nature of their mental illness, do not care for their own health and may damage or infect themselves or get injured in fights or suicide attempts.

From the beginning, treatment was educative. The patients were to learn self-control and better mixing socially. Delusions and hallucinations may not matter if the sufferer can ignore them sufficiently to behave politely and co-operate in work and play. If a new patient can learn to fit in with ward society he is beginning to improve, and may later be able to fit in also with the more exacting society at home. If he can manage the easy-going demands of regular work in the hospital, he may be able to progress to paid work outside. This social teaching was given by the nurses, as a part of the developing specialty of psychiatric nursing. The nursing contribution to the asylum was very important but often misunderstood and overlooked. This chapter examines it, and the following chapter will look at other components of treatment: the chaplain's moral therapy, the occupational therapy, and Mr Millar's emphasis – good food.

Discovery of psychiatric nursing

A severely mentally ill person may be very unpredictable in behaviour: restless, impossible to reason with, uninhibited in aggression when thwarted or frightened, incomprehensible in feelings and reactions. They consequently frighten those around them. The way of coping with this in the 18th and early 19th century was to meet violence with violence, overpower them, chain them up, even beat them to induce respect for authority. Once under restraint in this way they could be ignored or forgotten and the chains and handcuffs continued till they died.

The first demonstration of another way of coping came in Paris in the aftermath of the French Revolution. J. B. Pussin, a senior male attendant (nurse), and Philippe Pinel, a doctor in charge, liberated 40 patients from their bonds and chains in 1798, and showed that the patients responded well to compassionate firmness, especially if allowed plenty of exercise, and given some work to do. This liberation, begun at the Bicêtre and continued when they moved to the Salpetrière, made an international impression. It was developed and carried further at an asylum in Lincoln by Drs Gardiner Hill and Charlesworth, who by stages abolished restraints on patients until their asylum functioned perfectly well with none at all. Dr John Conolly went to see their work for himself just before he was put in charge of Britain's then largest asylum (1000 beds) at Hanwell, Middlesex, in 1839, and he proceeded to apply the methods of non-restraint and to publicise them to great effect. In essence, for violence was substituted friendliness, sympathy and concern for the individual. His book *Treatment of the Insane without Mechanical Restraints* (1856) summarises his own and later experience, and is worth quoting.

> "a man who for a week or two has been violently maniacal . . . who . . . has terrified his family, broken the furniture of his house or attacked the neighbours; or harangued the public and disturbed the streets, and resisted all control until overcome by the police. He comes to the asylum bound very tightly, sometimes hand and foot, or fastened in a strait waistcoat. He is still violent, but exhausted; he is flushed, feverish, thirsty; in appearance haggard and in manner fierce or sullen. His voice is hoarse with shouting. He is unwashed, unshaved, half starved. . . . His violence is still dreaded and he exhibits capricious proofs of remaining strength. . . . It is part of the non-restraint system to remember, whatever the state and circumstances of a newly admitted patient may be, that he comes to the asylum to be cured, or if incurable, to be protected and taken care of and kept out of mischief, and tranquillised; and that the strait-waistcoat effects none of these objects. Therefore, although the patients may arrive bound so securely as scarcely to be able to move, they are at once released from every ligature and bond and fetter that may have been imposed upon them. They appear generally to be themselves surprised at this proceeding; and for a time are tranquil, yet often distrustful and uncertain in their movements . . . (they are visited as soon as possible by a medical officer who assures them by a few kind words that no ill-treatment is any longer to be feared, and the actions which follow support this) – the patient is taken gently to the bathroom and has the comfort of a warm bath . . . carefully dried and has clean and comfortable clothing put on: he is then led to the

dayroom and offered good and well-prepared food. The very plates, and knife and fork, and all the simple furniture of the table are cleaner by far than what he has lately been accustomed to. . . . But the patient may be too much absorbed in delusions, or too much occupied by anger, or by fear alone to derive immediate benefit . . . this state will not last very long if no severity and no neglect are permitted. . . . The patients however are often merely restless or fidgety; run about; or are inclined to acts of harmless mischief. . . . One of the things which attendants are slowest to learn is not to interfere unnecessarily.''

At about the same time as Pussin and Pinel at the Salpetriere, George Jepson and Catherine Allen, the chief nurses at the Quaker private asylum, the Retreat at York, were introducing what came to be termed 'moral treatment', the psychological handling rather than the forcing of patients. As with Conolly it was concern for the individual. They tried to understand his or her feelings, tried to remedy grievances where possible, offered explanations of what was going on, tried to gain a person's confidence by offering affection. They tolerated 'bad' behaviour without rancour as an aspect of the illness, and tried to remain calm and understanding at all times. A patient thus won over by a nurse would usually try to behave in a socially acceptable way if only to please her. An observant nurse could recognise when a patient was beginning to get upset, and could distract him with a new interest or a change of occupation or a move to a less unfriendly seeming environment (e.g. going to bed for a few hours). The friendliness was emphasised by trying to furnish the hospital ward like a drawing room and holding afternoon tea parties and other group activities.

Dr Samuel Gaskell, when he became superintendent of Lancaster Moor Asylum in 1840 – the second largest in the country – at once began introducing non-restraint and the practices of moral treatment (ward psychotherapy, one might say) with great effect. He left in 1849 to become one of the three medical Commissioners in Lunacy in London, and in this capacity several times inspected the Bucks County Pauper Lunatic Asylum (1853–56). Lord Shaftesbury had by then been won over to the virtues of non-restraint, and so encouraged the abolition of all leg irons, handcuffs, chains and the like. Mr Millar was proud to report that his new asylum possessed no such equipment of any sort, and it is clear from his writings that he was a firm believer in moral treatment and non-restraint.

This beginning of psychiatric nursing was a distinctive British contribution to world psychiatry. W. Griesinger, the father of modern neuropsychiatry, Professor of Clinical Medicine and Mental Science at Berlin University, wrote in the second edition of his classic textbook (1861):

''Up to the time of the publication of the first edition of this work – influenced by the arguments of French and German psychologists – I opposed the system of non-restraint . . . since then, practical experience from the one end of England to the other has convinced me. I have seen with happy astonishment how easily several patients on the point of

> an outbreak were rendered speedily calm through a kind of psychical
> diversion, who to a certainty in the majority of Continental institutions
> would at once have had means of restraint applied.''

Unfortunately moral treatment and non-restraint lacked the glamour of
scientifically proved techniques, and were not widely publicised outside the
asylum world. Nor was there any formal teaching of them within that world,
because psychiatry was barely a distinct subject – it was to be picked up from
experience and private reading only. In consequence its practice depended
on those doctors already aware of it and able to teach it to the people they
appointed as nurses. As Gaskell soon found out, it was not easy to recruit
people of the right personality able to learn and practise as psychiatric nurses
(he did not call them that, of course), nor once trained would they necessarily
stay in the work. Yet contact with the same patients over many months
enabled a nurse to get to know them well as individuals, and so made the
work much easier. After Gaskell left Lancaster Moor the asylum slowly began
to revert to the old ways of restraint and bullying, though it never went
completely back. In the later 19th century the techniques were to an extent
generally forgotten.

It was not only the asylum staffs who found it difficult to carry on with
moral treatment, but the general public who remained unaware of it,
particularly that part of the public which governed the public asylums. They
had no conception of what psychiatric nursing could be, and saw the nurse
as part gaoler, part domestic servant. In consequence they were not going
to spend much money on nursing staff or on designing and furnishing their
asylums like middle-class homes when paupers were going to live there.
Conolly himself resigned from Hanwell in 1852 because his Committee
would not accept his advice on such broadly therapeutic matters. The
Commissioners in Lunacy tried to keep non-restraint and moral treatment
alive, but an annual inspection visit and occasional printed letters of advice
from London were not enough. In March 1859 they sent out a circular on
the personal qualities to be looked for in prospective nurses, some extracts
from which follow:

> "As regards Pauper Lunatics the Attendants should be capable of
> directing and promoting their occupations and amusements, of reading
> to them and of instructing them in their various trades and employments.
> Qualifications of a higher order, and a superior degree of education are
> required in Attendants upon Private Patients to whom they are
> necessarily to a certain extent companions. In this point of view it is
> very desirable that the Attendants should not have to perform duties
> of a menial nature such as belong more properly to domestic servants.''

> ". . . it is indispensable that they should be adequately paid and that
> they should be encouraged in a course of good conduct by a periodical
> advance in their wages. It is important also that they should be afforded
> regular opportunities for temporary absence and relaxation.''

"The experience and observation of the Commissioners leads them to believe that the above considerations have been to a great extent lost sight of in the selection and remuneration of Attendants."

Such considerations certainly did not remain within the view of the Bucks Committee.

Unfortunately restraint (equals neglect, said Conolly) is cheaper than other methods.

Early days at Stone

When the asylum opened in 1853, with five wards for men and five for women (see Table 3.2, p. 38), each ward had one nurse or attendant who lived in it, ate in it, and slept in it at night so as to be available for 24 hours. Time off amounted daily to two hours (8 p.m.–10 p.m.) except on one weekday when it began at 4 p.m. and one Sunday off in four. There was no annual leave, with or without pay. A night nurse was additionally provided only for the infirmary ward, to attend the physically sick. The total staff for up to 200 patients was therefore six men and a head male nurse, plus seven women, a needlewoman, and a matron (who was there partly as a chaperone). Apart from board and lodging the men earned £18 p.a. and the women £13–£15, the night staff a pound or so extra. This was more than the cook or three housemaids got. There were of course no ward maids, domestic assistants or clerical aids. The nurse : patient ratio might thus be put at 13 : 200 or 1 : 15, though for the first two years the asylum was not full. The staffing made no allowance for people being sick, or vacancies unfilled as soon as someone left, and the Commissioners were soon urging (without effect) the appointment of supernumerary nurses who could take over temporarily, or strengthen the ward staffing when there were several violent or suicidal patients in one ward.

The head nurses had previous asylum experience elsewhere, but the rest were mostly recruited locally from neighbouring villages or towns like Aylesbury and Oxford, and had worked in domestic service or as labourers or as artisans. Most were young, but one or two were married or widowed. The turnover was high – none taken on in 1853 were still there at the end of 1854. It took some years to achieve greater stability but by 1879 the Commissioners could note that only one male nurse out of 16 and four women out of 21 had been less than one year on the staff.

Local families began a regular habit of expecting to work "up at the mental", as they said in the 1920s. The earliest example was the Kemps. Richard joined as stoker in 1853, his mother joined as night nurse in January 1854, after one week's training at the asylum, and when Richard left his brother Thomas took his job. In November 1854 brother John began as night nurse, but soon changed to days, and sister Ann in February 1855. John resigned in July that year, and the rest of the Kemps resigned in August.

The male nurses' uniform is shown in Fig. 7.1.

Some of the work the staff did is displayed in the printed booklet *Regulations for the Attendants and Servants in the Pauper Lunatic Asylum of the County of Buckingham at Stone, near Aylesbury* (1876). The daily ward routine:

> "*6.00 am* All the attendants and servants to be dressed and ready for duty. The attendants to open the bedroom doors of such of the inmates as are fit to be at large. Any patient who appears in the slightest degree to be ill should be allowed to remain in bed until the Head Attendant comes round.
>
> *7.00 am* (in summer, 8.30 am in winter). Workers in the laundry to go there under the care of a laundress. Outworkers to go out with an attendant or gardener. The Stores required for the day will be delivered at the Kitchen.
>
> *8.00 am* Breakfast. Morning prayers to be read in each ward.
>
> *10.00 am* The medical visit on the male side shall commence: the wards are to be all cleaned, beds made, and everything in order by this time. On the female side the medical visit shall be made at 11 am. The Attendants are expected to be dressed in their uniform by this hour.
>
> *10.30 am* Dinner utensils to be left at the kitchen, when the lunch beer and extras ordered for the sick will be given out.
>
> *12.30 pm* Laundry and Outworkers return to dinner. The attendants shall see that they change their shoes, wash, and are tidy for dinner.
>
> *12.45 pm* Patients' dinner.
>
> *1.30 pm* Half of the attendants dine. Laundry workers return to work.
>
> *2.00 pm* The other attendants dine. Outworkers return to work.
>
> *2.30 pm* Attendants all on duty.
>
> *5.00 pm* Female patients to have tea.
>
> *5.30 pm* Outworkers leave work.
>
> *6.00 pm* Supper for male patients. 6.00–7.00 pm second medical visit.
>
> *7.00–8.00 pm* The patients go to bed. All the shutters to be locked, clothing removed from the rooms, doors locked, gas turned down, etc.
>
> *8.00 pm* The night attendants enter on their duty.
>
> *8.00–10.00 pm* Day attendants on leave. From 1 October to 31 March the gates are locked at 9.30 pm.
>
> *10.15 pm* All the attendants are expected to go to bed, and all lights not required by the night attendants to be extinguished.''

It will be noticed that the nurses were allowed only 30 minutes to eat their main meal of the day, and were ordered to bed at just after 10.00 p.m. The patients had to go to bed two or three hours earlier, and had at least ten hours in bed (otherwise more staff would have been required to supervise them). Their tea or supper was early and they then had to go about 14 hours, perhaps with an hour's work in the morning, before their next meal, breakfast.

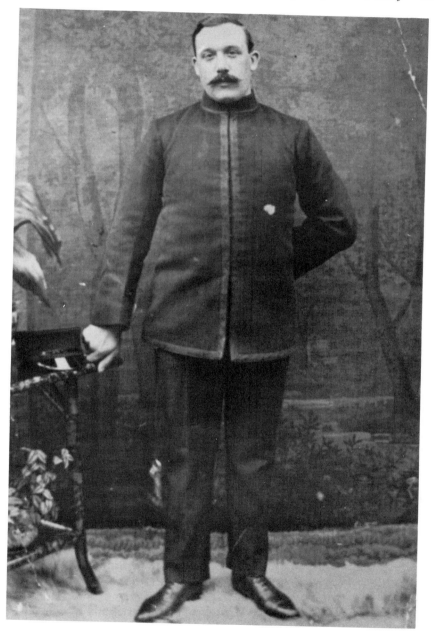

Fig. 7.1 The male nurses' uniform, before 1914

Some numbered regulations in the booklet enlarged on the nurses' routine:

"*No. 26*   At meal times the tables are to be prepared with order and regularity, and everything is to be ready before the patients take their seats. Grace is to be said before and after each meal by the attendant in charge of the ward, and the utmost order is to be maintained. The patients are not to be allowed to give their food to each other, nor remove any article from the table. Immediately after dinner the knives and forks are to be counted and carefully secured, and all utensils are to be restored to their places immediately after use. After breakfast and tea prayers are to be read in each ward by the attendant in charge. [It might have been added that some patients would require feeding, or having their food cut small for them.]

No. 22   The patients are to change their flannel [underwear] once a week and to have clean linen twice a week. Their beds and bedding are to be freely exposed to the air every morning for at least an hour.

No. 21   Every patient (unless prevented by illness) shall have a warm bath once a week in warm weather, and not less frequently than once a fortnight in cold weather (the temperature of the water marked on the thermometer is not to be less than 85 degrees (F) nor more than 96 degrees). On these occasions a careful examination is to be made of the body and an entry made in the daily returns if anything unusual be observed.''

A circular of 8 June 1857 from the Commissioners said a head attendant should be present throughout bath-time, to look for unreported wounds which could have resulted from ill-treatment. In 1859 they condemned the practice of bathing up to three patients in the same bath water, and still condemned it in 1870. The hot-water cisterns were too small to allow many baths per hour, and the staff could not afford the time to allow baths one at a time. The deficient and sometimes irregular water supply meant that at times baths were stopped for months, and also helped to slow the laundry, so that the recommendation of clean linen twice a week (1861) or two shirts a week for the men (1873) could not be followed. Suggestions that each patient should have a towel and toilet paper when required were councils of perfection.

Nurses had other duties also. They had to prepare the patients for divine service in the chapel on Sundays and Wednesdays, and for special occasions such as a visit by the Bishop. Groups of 20 to 50 patients were to be regularly taken out for country walks every week, with one nurse leading and another at the tail, taking care the male and female groups took different routes and did not meet. In the ward they were supposed to supervise and teach needlework, promote games and encourage reading, and of course continue housekeeping. They had hardly time for much befriending and understanding.

There were frequent comments on the understaffing in the Commissioners' reports of their annual inspections: "The majority of the patients sit listless and wholly unoccupied" (1875): "Number 6 ward with 45 noisy, destructive or demented patients had only 3 nurses, and better results might be obtained with more'' (1879); "Wards sometimes only have one attendant for 30 to 40 patients during part of the day'' (1880). A day nurse after a day's work sometimes also had to sit up at night, to help out. In 1879 the staff had grown to a total of 30 by day for about 480 patients (a ratio of 1 : 16). Back in 1870 the inspectors were already recommending the employment of women in some of the male wards, but this was never taken up until after 1945. The Committee, whether of magistrates or county councillors, was at all times very unwilling to expand the staff, the cost of which went on the bill of the parish or unions, which had to pay so much a week for their citizens who were patients. In the early days a nurse cost £15 in wages and £25 in keep, say, and £40 per year divided over 50 weeks and 200 patients comes to one penny per head per week for every extra nurse taken on. On a weekly cost of 9s 6d or 114 pence, one penny (or even five) does not seem a big increase, but the Committee was frightened of it.

Prevention of ill-treatment

The staff were reminded in the 1876 *Regulations* booklet that:

> "an asylum is a hospital for the treatment and cure of mental disease
> . . . and that the patients are irresponsible agents, visited in the all-
> wise providence of God with severe disease, and that the utmost
> forebearance is therefore to be exercised towards them. . . . However
> annoying the observations or conduct of the patients may be the
> attendants must regard it as evidence of a disordered mind, and they
> must be careful never to exhibit any appearance of anger or irritation,
> but should endeavour to treat all with uniform kindness."

> "*No. 28* Every attendant and servant will be liable to instant dismissal
> by the Superintendent, without further warning or notice, for being
> intoxicated, or for striking, ill-using or neglecting any of the patients
> (the wages of such attendants and servants being paid up to the day
> of dismissal)."

Section 123 of the Lunatic Asylums and Pauper Lunatics Act 1845 provided that abuse, ill-treatment or wilful neglect would be a misdemeanour chargeable at court.

The need for safeguards was indicated by the whole history of the private care of the mentally ill (1750–1850), and by the continuing abuses and scandals revealed from time to time in the asylums thereafter. A principal function of the Commission in Lunacy and its successor the Board of Control was to look out for abuse (and prosecute if necessary), and the inspectors aimed to encourage every patient to speak with them and complain of ill-treatment (though of course some might be too frightened to do so). Regular visiting of the asylums by members of the local Committee of Visitors was to look out for abuses, the Superintendent was to be on the watch also, and the head nurses. The day and night ward nursing reports, injury books, the daily hospital report, the seclusion book, and the Superintendent's journal were all written records of what was going on. If a patient was discovered to be injured (say at bath-time or at interview) and it was not explained or even mentioned in the ward reports beforehand, the ward staff would be held responsible. Of course, human loyalties being what they are, staff might combine to keep silent over abuses or the Committee keep them as internal secrets, ashamed and frightened of publicity. Hushing up, however, fails to discover why they have taken place. In a few cases it may be sadistic or perverted people indulging their tastes. More often neglect or harm to patients arises when nursing morale is low through bad management. The nurse is unsupported in her/his work, is given too much to do with too little aid, or asked to work for very long hours where extra pay cannot compensate for fatigue, feelings of injustice, and resentment. Not able to criticise and hit back at the management which is blithely indifferent to the problem, the nurse takes it out on the irritating or tedious patient instead. Unauthorised restraints, a beating to impose discipline, are shortcuts to lessen the work load as well as relieve feelings.

This said, the Bucks asylum appears to have been free of serious abuses. Over the decades 1853–1933 very few nurses appear to have been sacked for ill-treating patients, and there is only one record of an outside complaint. The inspectors year after year gave their impressions of good feeling and kindness between patients and staff, and said they never received any complaints of mishandling. No adverse reports have yet turned up, but even without them we must remain aware that inhumanity is endemic in institutions and may always reappear. Safeguards which work are always needed (see also Chapter 12).

The nurse's lot

The nursing staff's terms of service slowly improved. By 1870 they were being allowed annual leave, and from 1871, on the Commissioners' suggestion, were granted board wages while away. In 1880 came the proposal that pensions should be offered to those who had given long service, and the Committee began to grant them to the few individuals who had given 15 or 20 years to the asylum and were retiring through sickness or age. In 1909 came the Asylum Officers Superannuation Act which created regular contributory pensions, and the Committee raised wages slightly to enable staff to pay their contributions. The following year the Asylum Workers Union was founded, and its negotiations with the Mental Hospitals Association representing county councils as employers led in 1919 to a 60-hour working week with 30-minute breaks each day for breakfast, tea and dinner, two whole days off each week (and every third Sunday), and two weeks' annual leave in each six months. Artisan staff were to work a

48-hour week at union or district rates of pay (less one-sixteenth because of hospital privileges such as free meals at work), with bank holidays plus one week's annual leave with pay. This represented a great improvement for the nurses, and a recognition of their superior (professional) status. Conditions were to be further improved by national agreements in 1934, 1946 and later.

The new nurse learned patient and ward management on the job from colleagues of greater experience, guided to a certain extent by the doctor in special matters such as the care of epileptics. There was quite an amount of physical nursing to be done, not only of the partially paralysed or the tuberculous or those with diarrhoea, but of more acute conditions such as pneumonia or influenza, and a whole range of end-states from the common cardiac or renal failure to the rare special forms of cancer (see Table 9.8, p. 126). At Stone the infirmary wards were soon far too small for the number of physically sick, who consequently had to be nursed also in the ordinary wards, making it particularly necessary that all nurses could cope with physical problems. The Commissioners called for years for more infirmary accommodation, but to no avail.

With the development of medicine, surgery, and general nursing in the latter part of the 19th century, and the improvement of nursing employment in a professional direction, the doctors in charge of asylums began to feel that formal instruction of nurses was desirable. The Medico-Psychological Association produced a textbook of instruction in 1885. It was a 64-page booklet, but a new edition followed in 1893, and by the fifth edition in 1908 it was over 370 pages long, and criticised as having far too much anatomy and physiology and too little psychiatry. The Association also began in 1891 holding annual examinations for a Certificate in Attendance and Nursing upon Insane Persons (Fig. 7.2), which could only be taken after a two-year (later, three-year) course of compulsory lectures by the superintendent or his assistant, and clinical ward exercises by him or the head attendants. The examination was set centrally, but at first mounted locally – by Mr Humphry himself with an outside assessor such as Mr Sankey, the assistant from Littlemore who sometimes acted as his locum when he went on leave. By 1899 over 100 asylums were participating, and external examiners were being used, granting more than 500 certificates annually.

This training of mental nurses on a national scale began well before that of general nurses (the General Nursing Council (GNC) and state registration date from 1920) and continued distinct from it until the coming of the National Health Service. This helps to explain why for so long mental nurses stood somewhat apart from the rest of the nursing profession, and had their own union outside the Royal College of Nursing. Today most of this separation has gone. St John's was recognised by the GNC as a nurse training school in 1946. A proportion of nurses have double training (State Registered Nurse as well as Registered Mental Nurse) but there is still a proportion of nursing assistants and state enrolled nurses without any examinations passed (see p. 172).

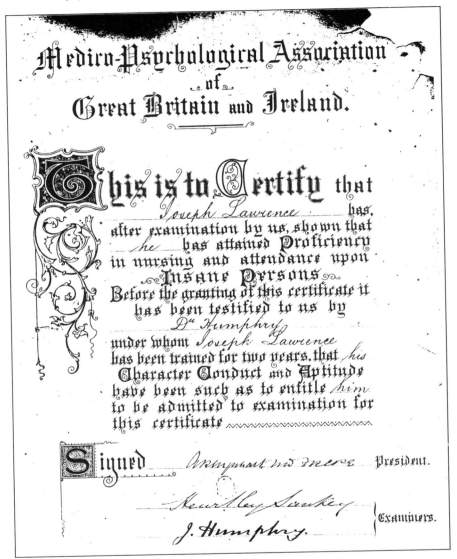

Fig. 7.2 The Nursing Certificate of 1891

Dr Kerr gave the teaching at Stone more or less from the time he arrived, and during the war years it was suspended. Thereafter the assistant Dr Mark Anthony had the job until 1934. Chapter 6 tells of the rigid invariant hierarchical asylum of 1890–1934, and the latter year brings us into the memory span of those still alive and able to describe their experience as nursing recruits in those days.

As they tell it, the new recruit was simply put on a ward on six months' probation, and picked up the routine of management from the next most junior nurse on the ward. It could be very hard work, with the risk of an occasional black eye. Some could not stand the feeling of being locked in. There was the endless jingle of keys, as each member of staff had a bunch of keys on a strong leather belt, and there was endless locking and unlocking. There was also endless counting of patients in and out, and of knives and forks before and after every meal. Each ward had its padded cell, its strong clothing and untearable mattresses. Patients were regularly searched. The various routines were supposed to give patients a feeling of security. The staff were supposed to entertain them, on and off the ward, and some discipline was maintained by threatening "you won't go to the football match unless you do so and so". Staff had all their meals on the wards, and were still on duty during meals. Living in was compulsory (unless married) and every one had to be in by 10 p.m. Even nurses were liable to be searched, and their baggage examined, whenever they left the hospital. Male and female staff were completely segregated (like the patients) and could not be seen together even when engaged to be married.

After the first year, the recruits had to attend 45-minute lectures in their own time. When Dr Mark Anthony was responsible he had a military approach, and would only stay ten minutes, then give the order "Open Chapter X [of the handbook] and carry on reading". Next time he would spend a few minutes asking questions. Male and female staff were taught separately, but the matron gave all the lectures on nursing. After 1934 Dr Tattersall came, and proper teaching began.

The doctors expected extremely respectful treatment. All staff had to stand to attention and salute them, and if the son of a staff member failed to touch his cap there was a reprimand. Even after 1945 a doctor complained to a senior nurse "I've never been so insulted in my life. Your nurse didn't stand up when I came on my round."

There was a social hierarchy in the hospital. The engineers were regarded as riff-raff and could only attend the Annual New Year's Dance with special permission. The laundresses could only attend if they wore their uniform. Artisan and labouring staff were on a different financial basis from those in contact with patients, as no sick pay and no pensions were allowed by the Committee. It was however possible to start as a bakery assistant or a housemaid and transfer to a nursing job, with its better pay and security.

Recruitment had its ups and downs – mostly the latter in the 20th century when local people could get work in the Oxford or Bedford/Luton automobile factories or work on the Rothschild estates. Many men who had served a while in the Army or Navy were glad to get into asylum service with its discipline. Ex-miners flocked into the mental hospital service after the General Strike in 1926 and the Depression of 1931. People who had something more than strength and discipline were favoured, perhaps an ex-bandsman, or a footballer or a theatrical worker, not only to help the

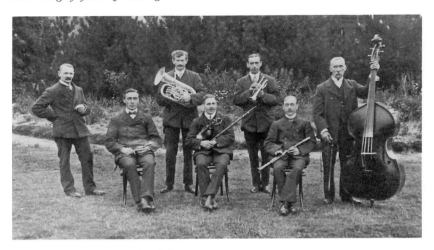

Fig. 7.3 The hospital orchestra in 1913

patients but contribute to the staff social life (the hospital orchestra is shown in Fig. 7.3). Women who at the beginning of the 20th century had little but domestic work open to them found their opportunities widening with factory work and office work during and after World War I, and by 1939 their recruitment to the mental hospital was getting more difficult. Girls from Wales, Ireland and the north-east of England substituted for locals.

Dr Skottowe, who created a revolution in so much, tried to improve the nurses' life with only a modicum of success. He largely failed to get proper accommodation for them, and a nurses' home remained a dream. Something of what happened after 1935 appears in Chapter 10; but the nursing problems and developments after 1950 have an extended discussion in Chapter 12.

Notes

Two sources of further reading regarding the introduction of kindly nursing are recommended:

DIGBY, A. (1985) *Madness, Morality and Medicine: A Study of the York Retreat 1796–1914*. Cambridge: Cambridge University Press.
HUNTER, R. & MACALPINE, I. (eds) (1973) *Treatment of the Insane without Mechanical Restraints* (by John Connolly, 1856). London: Dawson.

The source of the quote from Griesinger is:

GRIESINGER, W. (1861) *Mental Pathology and Therapeutics*. (Trans. C. Lockhart Robertson & J. Rutherford (1867). London: New Sydenham Society.)

8 Idle hands and empty stomachs

Organised religion in the form of the Anglican Church played a more important part in the treatment of psychiatric patients in England in the 19th century than it did thereafter. The asylum at its opening in 1853 had an integral chapel, and when the number of patients began to increase and expansion became necessary a bigger chapel was one of the first additions. The Commissioners on their inspection visits always inquired how many men and women were attending the services and frequently urged greater efforts to increase attendances. For the first 25 years the Committee of Visitors always seemed to have four or five Anglican clergy on it (about a third of the membership), and the Rev. Ouvry was Chairman 1869–86.

The chaplain, a non-resident, was paid like an assistant medical officer, one of the top salaries in the asylum, and was required to do much more than hold one or two services on Sundays. He had to visit all the wards frequently, talk with all the patients, read to them and pray with them, and keep a journal of all his activities to present for inspection at the monthly committee meetings. As the asylum expanded his pay rose from £80 per annum to £120 in 1872, and to £150 in 1876 when he had to hold an additional midweek service. He contributed his own section to the annual reports, though curiously separated from the reports of Chairman, Superintendent and inspectors by the statistics of the patients, but before the accounts. Those statistics showed that in most years about three-quarters of the patients admitted annually were Anglican, and the rest Methodist or Baptist with an occasional Roman Catholic or Quaker. They also in the early years attempted to list the moral or psychological causes of the attacks of madness leading to admission, suggesting that mental illness was not regarded as solely the preserve of the medical man at that time (Table 8.1).

The Rev. J. B. Reade, the vicar of Stone and a noted original photographer, astronomer, and eventually president of the Royal Microscopical Society, accepted to become the first chaplain when invited to do so. He stayed six years, resigning in 1859 when he moved to Ellesborough, a few miles away. In his last annual report he wrote:

TABLE 8.1
*Supposed causes of attack of mental illness, as recorded
in the annual report of 1854*

Cause	No. of patients
Males	
Grief, reverses	5
Grief, disappointment	1
Anxiety	3
Intemperance	8
Depraved habits	6
Fit	2
Fever	1
Age	1
Epilepsy	8
General paralysis	11
Congenital deficiency	8
Unknown	27
Total	27
Females	
Grief, seduction and desertion	3
Grief, loss of relatives	8
Grief, misconduct of children	2
Grief, disappointed affection	4
Grief, domestic misery	5
Grief, desertion by husbands	2
Anxiety about business	1
Anxiety about child	1
Altercation with neighbour	1
Fright	3
Remorse	1
Religious enthusiasm	1
Fever	3
Injuries to head	1
Loss of blood	1
Intemperance	2
Severe illness	1
Age	1
Epilepsy	7
General paralysis	2
Congenital deficiency	9
Unknown	48
Total	110
All patients	
With relatives known to be insane	66
With suicidal tendency	
male	11
female	13
With deafness	
male	3
female	8

"I seldom fail to receive from newly-admitted patients, when not absolutely unimpressible and obstinately silent, some account of the state of their minds as well as of the causes which led to their illness. The most common causes are religious melancholy, loss of health, loss of property, and drunkeness. I have given such advice and reproof as the cases seemed to require, and generally the reproof was well received and richly deserved."

The next year, the Rev. Charles Lowndes (vicar of Hartwell) wrote:

"Although I have stated that the patients are generally attentive, it must not be supposed that all who attend Chapel worship God in spirit and in truth, far from it. Still the hope may be indulged that even these may derive some degree of benefit from what they hear; and, besides, we cannot doubt that the self-control which they are compelled to exercise while there, must have a beneficial effect upon them. There are however a few cases of melancholia upon whom religion seems not to have any effect, and who give themselves up entirely to despair, being tormented with the delusion that they already feel the flames of Hell. Such cases it is painful to witness. But I may add, on the other hand, that there are others also, who far from dreading any punishment in the next world, appear perfectly happy and contented, and when questioned as to their prospects of the future say that they feel quite satisfied on that point; a few even fancy themselves already in Heaven."

The Rev. Lowndes continued to serve until his road accident in 1880, when the Rev. C. Ridley of Aylesbury took over till 1904. There followed a succession of curates doing two-year stints – Challis, Holbrooke, Edwards – suggesting a certain downgrading in the importance of the post. From 1910 the Rev. Stukely provided continuity, though it is noteworthy that after 1916 there were no further notes from the chaplain in the annual reports. The later reports had been less confident that anything worthwhile was being achieved by the religious activity. I have not been able to determine exactly how the role of religion declined, but it did, as in society at large.

By 1923 both a Nonconformist minister and a Roman Catholic priest were listed as additional visiting chaplains, and eventually they also were allowed to hold an occasional service in the chapel. There was no longer the idea of offering religious therapy to all, but help only to believers ready to accept it.

Occupations

The importance of giving patients something to do while they were in the asylum was not recognised by the local planners of 1850. No allowance for work rooms or storage cupboards was made in the design of the original building, the grounds were seen as areas of recreation, the early equipment was of games and pastimes. However, under Mr Millar men began to be employed as helpers in the gardens and on the farm, and women in the

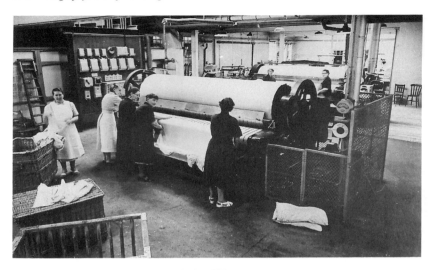

Fig. 8.1 Patients at work in the laundry in the 1930s

laundry (Figs 8.1, 8.2) while many women in the wards sat sewing dresses and curtains and the like for the asylum. The Commissioners in Lunacy urged that the patients should cover all their daily needs of boots and shoes and clothing and bedlinen by their own work, but this was seen more in terms of economy than benefit to the individuals concerned, and therefore employed the docile coherent patients and not the disturbed and mentally or physically weaker. The employment offered reflected the world outside

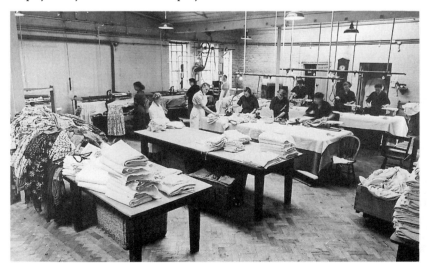

Fig. 8.2 Patients at work in the ironing room in the 1930s

the asylum. Women were accustomed to all kinds of domestic tasks, and men in a rural county predominantly worked on the land. Nevertheless, never more than 10% of the male patients at most were ever thus employed.

Year by year the annual reports record in detail the production of clothes and linen. Table 8.2 gives some of what was reported for 1868 and 1913.

The trouble was that the range of occupations on offer was limited, employment went to those who already knew how to do that work, and to the more co-operative and energetic. Often the Commissioners commented at their visits on the numbers of patients sitting listless and unoccupied, and eventually deteriorating through boredom and the deadening routine of the day.

Occupation not only might prevent boredom and deterioration but had positive benefits to offer. It could help to distract patients' thoughts from their symptoms and illness, it could build up their shattered self-confidence and help them in social relations; to the staff it was a test to measure the extent of a patient's recovery. In Germany, notably at Gutersloh near Hanover, where Dr Simon was a pioneer at the start of the 20th century, arts and handicrafts were offered and taught to the patients – drawing and painting and music groups, carpentry and iron work, pottery and working with glass, raffia and cane work, embroidery. The emphasis was on activity to benefit and develop the patient, not to produce a saleable product, though eventually the better products came to be offered for sale on stalls at the gates of some Continental asylums.

The development of occupational therapy passed by the Bucks County Mental Hospital until after World War II (see p. 81). The Committee, like many others, had its eye on money and was uncomprehending. It was this which led the Ministry of Health in the late 1950s to decide to recommend the closure of all hospital farms. They had become of ever less value to the patients as Britain became more and more industrialised and technological, and they distracted Committee members and hospital management with the promise of profits remote from the prime purposes of the hospital. The farm at St John's Hospital was closed in 1962, and the land let to local farmers.

TABLE 8.2
Some annual clothing production figures

	1868 (115 women patients)	1913 (370 women patients)
Gowns (dresses)	298	421
Chemises	257	300
Flannel vests	96	150
Petticoats	105	106
Shirts	158	293
Sheets	175	465
Bolster cases	125	419

In 1913 the tailor produced 274 jackets and 397 pairs of trousers, and the shoemaker made all the boots, shoes and slippers for the hospital.

The development of occupational therapy after World War II

Occupational therapy required space, and it needed special staff. When Peveril Court and the wartime huts in its grounds were purchased in 1946, two of the huts were moved to the hospital grounds to become an occupational therapy department and two posts for therapists were established – young women who had received a special training which combined art and handicraft teaching with some knowledge of medicine, and encouraged them to be inventive in what they offered patients. In the course of time discussion groups, gymnastics to music, dancing and drama were added. Two therapists were not enough for the full needs of the hospital, and their work was not greatly valued by some of the medical staff, who thought of it as a hobby for women patients – for those who enjoyed embroidery or making mats from plaited straws. In consequence the therapists felt neglected and discouraged and did not stay very long. Sometimes there was only one; eventually there were none. The nurses tried to bridge the gap to some extent, and for a time the local education authority was willing to send in adult-education teachers in handicraft and art.

Of course enormous changes in way of life took place after 1946. Many patients spent only a few weeks or months in hospital, and during at least part of that time were going home on leave regularly, so that boredom and hopelessness were less. Radio and television became available in all wards, and washing machines for patients' use in some of them. The hospital laundry could be dispensed with, as a specialist would take the soiled linen and bring back the fresh. Clothes of good design and low price were being offered by Marks and Spencer and other stores, and for patients who could not go to the shop themselves a store would stage a dress show at the hospital. The old occupations for women in laundry and in dressmaking had gone. The coming of do-it-yourself to the home meant that men in hospital could undertake redecorating and repairs, although workers' unions were concerned about the possible loss of jobs by their members, and their representatives had difficulty in understanding that being sick is not necessarily a reason for being off work (quite the reverse, sometimes).

But a new range of occupations for patients emerged in 'industrial therapy'. It had begun in Bristol, where a group of long-stay patients operated a (paying) car-wash service; it spread to the concept of short-term profitable contracts for a variety of services and manufacturing, such as packaging of hooks into plastic bags, ready for sale in the shops, printing tickets or small advertising leaflets, finishing small decorative chromium strips for Ford cars, and so on. The patients who worked were paid according to their work, but only up to a still small sum, so that they avoided income tax, national insurance and so on (they still had free board and lodging if they were in the hospital), and most of the profits went into a special fund for helping patients in general, and some of course into buying small machines for the factory.

Run by male nurses, industrial therapy began at St John's in 1958, and a special light spacious brick building was opened for it in 1962. During those first four years £11 500 was earned from such tasks as 13 250 indoor aerials made and packed, 300 teddy bears assembled, 44 000 labels stuck on matchboxes, 39 500 tubular chairs made and packed, over 2 million lipstick cases put together. Within the one building groups of patients worked on different projects, selected according to the patient's capacity. While the best might be working full days and hard, other patients might be capable of only a few hours or a very slow tempo of work – but all were in principle acceptable. An environment was provided in which people could gradually accustom themselves to the discipline and routine of work; for some it was a rehabilitation after long unemployment through illness.

The positive aim in the 1960s and 1970s was that no patient should have nothing to do, and that the wards should be empty during working hours. The nurse's old role as exerciser and entertainer had faded away, and the new roles were as occupation planner for the week, initiator of group activities, and psychotherapist. Women's health-and-beauty classes were introduced, a branch of the Women's Institute established, and so on, activities started by nurses but then carried on largely by patients. Ward discussion groups became common, sometimes dealing with ward administration, sometimes with symptoms and behaviour. The rapid changes in the nature of the work meant that staff needed further education and retraining. Groups of nurses were released from ward duties for a study day or seminars and lectures, to hear about the new drugs, or behaviour therapy, or new practical methods. Sometimes this was in hospital, sometimes at a regional centre or in London, which enabled mixing of staff from different hospitals, exchange of views and lessening of the isolation which in earlier days had been such a problem.

Food

John Millar at the start in 1853 remarked that many lunatics were underweight, and that therefore a good diet could hardly be bad treatment. But there were other ideas in the 19th century. J. C. Drummond and Ann Wilbraham in *The Englishman's Food* (1939) describe (p. 433) how the Poor Law Commissioners favoured ''a low diet'' because food ''too rich and exciting for indoor employment'' might result in lethargy or nervous ailments; and (p. 440) in prisons an excessive diet might provoke the poor to further crimes. As for lunatics, some laymen suspected they might well be easier to manage if weakened by semi-starvation. But as the century went on there was increasing evidence that underfed prisoners simply could not manage hard physical work, and that the malnourished inmates of institutions of all sorts became much more prone to infections and liable to die.

Scientific studies showed that an adult needed a certain minimum daily intake of protein and calories to avoid losing weight and becoming enfeebled. At the start of the 20th century it was realised that the quality as well as the simple quantity of protein mattered, and in the second decade the importance of vitamins for physical health came to the fore. The bleeding and sometimes fatal disease of scurvy had long been known to ships' companies, army units, and institutions. The lack of vitamin C which caused it could be corrected with lemon juice, potatoes and fresh fruit and raw green vegetables, and fresh milk. Lack of sufficient nicotinamide, one of the B vitamins, in institutional diets, notably in the southern USA and in Italy, gave rise to pellagra, in which mental symptoms were often prominent or even predominant. The controlled dietary of the Victorian asylum ran the risk of weakening the long-stay inmates in various ways, leading to new mental symptoms, physical illnesses and death. But in the earlier years necessary knowledge of nutrition was lacking, although falling bodyweights, epidemics, and death rates might offer hints to the observant.

The asylum or hospital committee for many years published annually a dietary for patients and for resident staff (Table 8.3). One can examine it for changes officially made over the years. Patients and staff received different allowances of meat, bread, vegetables and milk, and this comparison is useful as an expression of local opinion about suitable food for lunatics. One can work out roughly what a weekly diet might provide on average in terms of calories, minerals, etc. But such dietaries are pious hopes rather than realities. They are subject to availability of foodstuffs and to catering management on the one hand (including the extent to which the common kitchen favours the resident staff at the expense of the patients), and to the care with which patients eating in common are supervised on the other. Patients do not necessarily eat what is put before them; the strong may steal from the weak, the charitable give to the needy, quite apart from lack of appetite or dislike of what is offered. A nurse in charge of 30 or more disturbed people will be hard put to see that everyone gets their proper food allowance.

We have two other indicators of diet. The Commissioners in Lunacy (later the Board of Control) on their surprise annual visits made a point of seeing dinner served and noting what it was. In fact the reports are few. More usefully, the asylum annual reports contain accounts with lists of the quantities of various foods bought in the year, and the prices paid, which enable some very rough calculations to be made.

Overall, the dietary appears to have been fairly steady and adequate over the first 36 years of the asylum's existence, food costing £13–£15 per head per annum or about 5–6 shillings per week during a long period when prices were steady.

But the coming of the Bucks County Council changed all that from 1890. One of their first acts was to cut the weekly cost of maintenance from about 9 shillings to about 7 shillings per head, and most of this was a saving on food.

TABLE 8.3

The "ordinary diet table", reproduced from the annual report of 1865

	Breakfast					Dinner							Supper					
	Bread: ounces	Butter: ounces	Sugar: ounces	Tea: pints	Milk: pints	Roast meat: ounces	Boiled meat: ounces	Stew: ounces	Currant pudding: ounces	Vegetables: ounces	Bread: ounces	Beer: pints	Bread: ounces	Cheese: ounces	Beer: pints	Tea: pints	Butter: ounces	Sugar: ounces
Sunday																		
males	6	½	½	1	–	6	–	–	–	12	4	½	6	2	½	–	–	–
females	5	½	½	1	–	5	–	–	–	12	4	⅜	5	–	–	1	½	½
Monday																		
males	6	½	½	1	–	–	6	–	–	12	4	½	6	2	½	–	–	–
females	5	½	½	1	–	–	5	–	–	12	4	⅜	5	–	–	1	½	½
Tuesday								Stew										
males	6	½	½	1	–	–	–	16	–	–	6	½	6	2	½	–	–	–
females	5	½	½	1	–	–	–	12	–	–	5	⅜	5	–	–	1	½	½
Wednesday																		
males	6	½	½	1	–	–	–	–	16	–	–	½	6	2	½	–	–	–
females	5	½	½	1	–	–	–	–	12	–	–	⅜	5	–	–	1	½	½
Thursday																		
males	6	½	½	1	–	–	6	–	–	12	4	½	6	2	½	–	–	–
females	5	½	½	1	–	–	5	–	–	12	4	⅜	5	–	–	1	½	½
Friday																		
males	6	½	½	1	–	–	6	–	–	12	4	½	6	2	½	–	–	–
females	5	½	½	1	–	–	5	–	–	12	4	⅜	5	–	–	1	½	½
Saturday								Meat pie										
males	6	½	½	1	–	–	–	16	–	12	–	½	6	2	½	–	–	–
females	5	½	½	1	–	–	–	12	–	12	–	⅜	5	–	–	1	½	½

Stew to consist of 3 oz of meat and 13 oz of vegetables and herbs.

Currant pudding to consist of: 8 oz of flour, 2 oz of currants, and 2 oz of suet for males; 6 oz of flour, 1½ oz of currants, and 1½ oz of suet, for females.

Female patients employed in the laundry and kitchen, ¼ of a pint of ale with bread and cheese for lunch, 1 pint tea and 4 oz bread and butter at 4 o'clock p.m.

Male patients employed in the garden and in-door work, ½ pint of ale extra, with bread and cheese, at 11 o'clock a.m., and at 4 o'clock p.m.

Male attendants' and servants' weekly allowances, 2 oz tea, 4 oz coffee, 2 oz tea, 4 oz coffee, 16 oz Derby cheese, and 3½ pints new milk.

Female attendants' and servants' weekly allowances, 2 oz tea, 4 oz coffee, 8 oz fresh butter, 12 oz sugar, 16 oz Derby cheese, and 3½ pints new milk.

Male and female attendants and servants, 1¼ lb of bread daily, and dinner provided in male and female mess-rooms.

Male attendants, 2 pints ale each daily. Female attendants and servants, 1 pint ale each daily. Gardeners and lodge-keeper, 2 pints of ale each daily.

Thereafter for many years they boasted annually that the weekly maintenance cost was always one shilling less than the average cost for all the asylums of the whole country. They were proud to be among the cheapest of perhaps 100 institutions. When World War I came and prices began to rise, they cut food again to try to hold maintenance costs down. There was no official food rationing till 1918, but they imposed their own ration, and it was quite inadequate. The result was that the annual death rate among the patients began to rise year by year, reaching the astonishing figure of 257 (one-third of the patients) in 1918, mostly before the influenza epidemic of that autumn (which resulted in only 22 deaths of patients). With peace, the patients began to be weighed quarterly, at the insistence of the Board of Control, and instead of losing weight many of them began to gain a little. This coincided with a change of policy, a succession of dietary improvements, and a sudden leap allowed in weekly maintenance cost, from about 15 shillings per head in 1918 to 25 shillings per head in 1919. Thereafter food never appears to have been a serious issue. In World War II there was no excess of deaths or indication of malnutrition.

About 300 people, young as well as old, died unnecessarily during 1914–18 in the asylum, thanks to the meanness and ignorance of the county councillors. The details of the deaths are discussed in the following chapter. Here is simply offered some evidence about the food, firstly from the reports on the main meal of the day given by the visiting Commissioners.

> "11 Nov 1872
> Meat and vegetables, good and abundant.
> 6 Nov 1876
> Beef, potatoes and greens, bread and beer – tasted.
> 16 Oct 1886
> Meat 5 days a week, Thursdays Currant Pudding; today – damson pie with substantial crust, and beer or porter of good quality.
> 13 Jan 1892
> Sorry to find the diet worse: bacon in place of fresh meat one day a week, beer abolished except for workers. Today's soup appears less nutritious. (Steward explained they were running out of their carrots and onions.)
> 13 June 1893
> Meagre dinner of watery soup and bread – unpalatable and insufficient.
> 6 June 1896
> 'Rhubarb tart and water' was the full dinner.
> May 1905
> Soup and bread only for dinner: could not at least bread and cheese be added?''

In contrast:

> "29 Oct 1923
> Today dinner consisted of roast mutton, vegetable and potatoes followed by rice pudding. The food was of good quality, sufficient in quantity and cleanly served.

9 April 1924
I saw a good and substantial dinner of boiled bacon with potatoes, carrots
and bread . . . I am glad to see that improvements of a wide-ranging
character have been carried out recently, as regards the breakfast and
tea; on two days of the week butter is given in place of margarine, and
only one day of the week is margarine given without jam or cake for tea.''

Previously, in 1921, it was noted that porridge was added for breakfast and
a light supper was now being given in the evening; and one additional good
suet pudding per week was added.

Table 8.4 compares the weekly allowances of certain foods to male staff
and male patients in 1916 (women always had less). Very roughly, the staff
got officially at least four times as much protein and twice as many calories
as the patients, and their diet was not so very different from what it had
been in 1886. In that year the patients had less than the staff, but not so
very much less. By 1916 patients' meat was cut by about 30% and their
bread by 50% and they had lost their beer, which provided extra calories
and vitamins. One can calculate roughly the patients' daily allowance in
1916 of protein and calories: about 40 g protein and 750 calories (900 calories
if all the vegetable were potato). The minima for a sedentary adult man
are taken now to be not less than about 60 g protein and 2100 calories, so
it is obvious that the diet had become grossly deficient in calories. When
we compare the asylum's expenditure in 1889 and in 1892 on meat and
total provisions for the year, before and after the County Council's cut, we
can see that less and cheaper meat accounted for a good deal of the drop
in maintenance cost on 450 patients (Table 8.5).

It was known from the beginning of asylum days that some severely
mentally ill people refused all food, and even all drink, and that this could
be life-threatening. Compulsory feeding was therefore practised by passing

TABLE 8.4
Weekly food for men (patients and staff)

	Staff		Patients	
	1886	1916	1916	1886
Meat: oz	?	112	27	37
Bacon: oz	16	24	5	–
Bread: oz	140	112	48[1]	106
Butter: oz	8	7	3½	7
Sugar: oz	12	16	3½	–
Cheese: oz	16	16	1[2]	–
Milk: pints	3½	3½	some in tea	–
Vegetables[3]: oz	?	?	48	76

1. Patients were said to be allowed extra bread at dinner if they asked for it.
2. Working patients got extra bread and cheese at 11 a.m. on work days.
3. If all vegetables were potato at 23 cal/oz, 48 oz weekly = 160 cal daily.
Note that in 1916 staff got 136 oz animal protein weekly (excluding cheese), patients 32 oz, a fourfold
difference; staff got twice as much bread.
From the offical dietaries published in the annual reports. 1 oz = 28 g.

TABLE 8.5
Some annual food costs, 1889 and 1892

| | 1889 | | 1892 | |
	Weight: lb	Cost: £	Weight: lb	Cost: £
Australian meat	5880	111	6568	93
Beef and mutton	76187	2040	38451	949
Bacon	4645	126	1343	67
Total cost of provisions		5185[1]		3451[2]
Total cost per head per week[3]		4s 4d		3s 0d

1. With beer.
2. Without beer.
3. Saving of 1s 0d per week on meat alone over 1889–92.
There were about 450 patients in both years.

a tube from the mouth into the stomach and pouring in water or milk, or raw egg beaten in milk. Quite often after a day or two of this the patient would begin eating and drinking a little in the normal way, but if not tube-feeding would continue, because the alternative could be death.

As early as 1926 the practice of serving no food after 5 p.m. until breakfast next day had been criticised. In the late 1940s studies were published showing that where food was available at 7 p.m. and hot milk perhaps at 10 p.m. the patients slept very much better and it was possible to do without the hypnotics given out so freely each night. The saving on the drug bill was more than matched by the extra expense of keeping catering staff on duty after 5 p.m., but there is no doubt it is better practice.

Medical work

Since 1950 mental illness has become increasingly a medical matter, and not only because of the empirical discovery of some effective drugs. The growth of nutritional knowledge has shown that mental illness can result from vitamin deficiency, or poisoning by metals, while hormonal disturbances can act likewise in other cases. Closer study of many physical conditions is revealing that some of these can bring about brain changes leading to mental breakdown. The need for the doctor and the pathological laboratory is much greater than it was even 50 years ago.

However, the doctor was also needed in 1853. People who attempt suicide may need sewing up or washing out, those who have a severe mental illness are sometimes self-neglectful and therefore liable to infections more than other people – pneumonia, tuberculosis, dysentery – or acquire fractures or bedsores. Epilepsy and general paralysis of the insane are medical conditions, and mental illness following childbirth probably likewise. Alcoholism has many medical features. Patients might be admitted in the last stages of chronic bronchitis, or partially paralysed, or (to take cases from the

Superintendent's journal of 1878) suffering from carbuncle, hydatid cyst (due to a parasite) of liver, gangrene of the leg, chronic lupus, enlarged heart, and kidney failure. The asylum doctor had to face more medical and surgical illness than a general practitioner with the same size list of patients, and with much less opportunity to call in specialist aid until the last 60 years.

Notes

How little was spent on 'surgery and dispensary' or drugs each year is shown in the published annual accounts:

Year	No. of patients	Total cost	Salaries and wages	Drugs
1853	c. 200	£4034	£1028	£19
1886	c. 400	£12 102	£2973	£84
1902	c. 500	£11 294	£3570	£110
1926	c. 700	£64 296	£16 925	£261

Staff represent roughly a quarter of the total expense; drug expenditure rises from about ½% of total to nearly 1%, but drops below ½% of total in 1926. No account in the above is taken of the number of patients passing through the hospital in a year, and this figure greatly expanded after 1936, while the use of psychotropic drugs began after 1955.

The discovery of the importance of the vitamin nicotinamide for mental health by researchers in the 1920s is well described in:

SHEPHERD, M. (1978) Epidemiology and clinical psychiatry. *British Journal of Psychiatry*, **133**, 289–298.

9 What was the use?

The asylum was planned and opened in 1853 with the idea that it was to be a curative establishment, and patients would only stay a few months. This idea had some, but insufficient, basis in fact. Dr Hitch of the Gloucester Subscription and County Asylum had noted that over 50% of his patients (493 out of 917) between 1823 and 1838 had been discharged. The stay was only a matter of months in some small private institutions. It was supposed that catching the illness early would make cure easier, and the bulk of the observed recorded cases in fact had very short histories because, as we now can see, they were manic–depressives who were sent to hospital quickly and soon got better spontaneously, wherever they were (see Case 3 in Chapter 1, p. 8).

The first shock to the curative idea at Stone was the admission of patients who shortly after died; the second was more profound – the appearance of considerable numbers of incurable chronic sick whose existence had not been suspected. The magistrates began sending in the partially paralysed, the deaf and blind, the physically incapacitated and unemployed, the old and the young without family to care for them, provided they showed some behavioural disturbance as well. The workhouses were discouraged from taking them, or glad to get rid of them, and the charitable and private hospitals were too few and far between to accept them (or too costly). Indeed, even in the National Health Service of the last 30 years, provision for the chronic physically sick has been inadequate, and the psychiatric hospitals have helped to house them.

The functions discharged by the asylum and the mental hospital have changed over the decades as the kinds of patients sent to them have changed. This has been decided partly by family opinion, by community beliefs, by the actions of magistrates and other lay officials, aided and abetted from time to time by general practitioners and lawyers. But the illnesses of the population have changed also. Improvement in public health and the drop in infant mortality in the last quarter of the 19th century have affected the number of the mentally ill. The Committee which managed the asylum, and their medical superintendents before 1935, do not seem to have stopped to debate what the asylum was doing, supposedly or in fact. What was it for? It was taken as self-evident: the law said a building must be put up and maintained for lunatics, and the Committee would do this; what went on inside it was a matter for the doctors. The Committee would finance the fabric, the equipment, the delivery of consumables such as coal, hay and flour, but the doctors would dispose of the human beings also delivered there, as they thought fit. There was no idea that decisions taken about the building or the food or the size of the nursing and medical staff could modify the human outcomes. Yet the very existence of the asylum, bringing many people close together, created new dangers of death from dysentery or tuberculosis. The outcomes could be said to measure the success of the asylum and justify its cost. Nothing was put into words, or discussed, although it is instructive to do so now.

The sorts of people admitted

Up till 1931 all the inmates were lunatics, all on some kind of certificate ordering them in and the asylum or hospital to take them. But the term 'lunatic' covered a great diversity of ages and conditions (Table 9.1). Some might be children as young as six, others old people arriving for the first time at age 65 or even 80. Some were mentally handicapped from birth, others had a mental illness, which once started might either then be everlasting or of a kind which disappeared spontaneously in a few months. Delirium tremens (usually caused by interruption of alcoholic excess) remits in a few days.

Some illnesses were long recognised to be caused in some way by alcohol, others seemed to follow childbirth. General paralysis of the insane (GPI)

TABLE 9.1
Diagnoses of patients admitted in 1868

	Males	Females	Total
Mania, recent and acute	14	32	46
Mania, chronic	4	4	8
Mania, with epilepsy	1	2	3
Mania, with paralysis	0	2	2
Mania, with general paralysis	6	0	6
Mania, puerperal	0	2	2
Mania, recurrent	0	2	2
Melancholia	4	7	11
Dementia	4	1	5
Dementia, with epilepsy	1	2	3
Dementia, with paralysis	0	1	1
Congenital imbecility	2	3	5
Idiocy	0	3	3
Totals	36	61	97

NB Mania does not have its modern meaning.

was recognised at the end of the 19th century as a late result of syphilitic infection, and after about 1920 began to be treatable. Then there were many epileptics who also began to be treatable: they comprised a sixth of the asylum population in 1861 (see Table 5.2, p. 62); by 1961 it was hard to find one in hospital. The growth of railways, of motor traffic, especially motorcycles, led to accidents with many head injuries permanently damaging brains and a new need for long-term care.

Schizophrenia is often regarded publicly as the most typical of the asylum illnesses. In reality it was only one kind among a number, and difficult to put an exact figure to, because the diagnostic term belongs to the 20th century and patients earlier were classified differently and not always very thoroughly described. It is hard for us now to be sure what their trouble really was. Very roughly in Bucks today there is about one new schizophrenic patient each year in every 10 000 people. If this were so in the 19th century one would expect about 15–20 new cases a year. If none of them went to the workhouse and all came to the asylum it would still amount to only a quarter of the year's intake (see Table 9.3) of patients, and the number retained longer than one year fluctuated considerably but perhaps averaged about 15. The actual numbers are so small it is not possible to see any trend through the half-century. The great growth in the numbers in the asylum was more due to the senile and the mentally handicapped, and to greater longevity, than to increase in schizophrenia.

So the asylum played a variety of roles from the beginning. Firstly it was protective of the lunatic. It could provide a neutral environment away from the stresses of home and work and without responsibilities, which could favour recovery. Secondly, it relieved families of what could be a very heavy burden over many months, caring for a mentally sick relative, and offered a haven for the orphan and the solitary old person who could not manage. Thirdly, it provided some education and training, not only in living a social life tolerant of others and orderly, but at some times helped the illiterate, taught trades and hobbies, and encouraged music and drama. Fourthly, it provided a protective home for the incurable, and physical nursing for the ill and the dying. Fifthly, in the 20th century, it began to offer improved symptomatic and even fairly specific treatments for some conditions (Table 9.2). Of course it often performed these functions very poorly; this was human failure.

After 1931 people began to come in without certification, of their own free will, because they wanted treatment, and this led to many people coming who would never have been certifiable and therefore never admitted previously: people with depressive illnesses, severe neuroses, and so on. Ultimately they swamped the original psychotic, the 'mad', who became only a minority of the total, at times neglected or overlooked altogether in plans for mental health services.

Sampling some of the asylum/hospital statistics of admission and discharge, at ten-year intervals in Table 9.3 and at four-year intervals in most of

TABLE 9.2
Years of introduction of new treatments in psychiatry

Treatment	Year of introduction
Drugs	
Sedatives and hypnotics	
bromides	1857
chloral	1869
paraldehyde	1882
sulphonal	1888
barbital	1903
Antidepressants	
imipramine	1957
monoamine oxidase inhibitors	1957
Anti-epileptics	
phenobarbital	1912
phenytoin	1938
primidone	1953
carbamazepine	early 1960s
benzodiazepines	1968
Antipsychotics	
chlorpromazine	1953
haloperidol	1958
Techniques	
Malaria for GPI	1917
Continuous narcosis	1922
Insulin 'shock'/coma	1935
Metrazol convulsant	1935
Electroconvulsive therapy	1938
Leucotomy	1936–42
Psychological techniques	
hypnosis (Bernheim)	1884
catharsis (Janet)	1889
psychoanalysis (Freud)	1909
analytical psychology (Jung)	1913
group therapy	1946
behaviour therapy	1960
family therapy	1970

The dates are approximate only.

Table 9.4 will show how the intake varied importantly from time to time. The proportion of old people (over 60s) among the newcomers was around one-fifth in 1861–81, dropped to a sixth in 1891, and thereafter rose to a quarter of the total annual intake. They formed a part of the sudden rise in admissions following the Lunacy (Consolidation) Act 1890. Another part of this rise was in the numbers of mentally handicapped over 1891–1911. The summary for 1911 in the footnote to Table 9.3 shows that the physical nursing of the elderly and the care of mentally handicapped children had become important elements of the asylum's function, and we record elsewhere the persistent failure to provide adequate infirmary wards for nursing patients in bed, or a separate ward, and some education for the children shut up with adults. It was only after a number of avoidable deaths

TABLE 9.3

Annual admissions and discharges, 1861–1911

	1861	1871	1881	1891	1901	1911
Admissions						
Total	79	78	96	157	112	198
No. of Bucks patients admitted	63	71	87	108	108	193
No. (%) aged over 60	17 (21.5%)	17 (21.5%)	18 (18.7%)	22 (14%)	26 (24%)	47 (24%)
No. of epileptics	8	4	12	16	14	7
No. of mentally handicapped	4	2	4	9	10	22
First attack	50	69	71	132	91	127
Not first attack	29	9	23	25	21	48
Discharges						
No. discharged	32	51	31	58	45	81
No. who died	18	38	47	46	61	77
No. (%) dead in less than one year	5 (6%)	13(16%)	17 (18%)	16 (10%)	14 (12%)	23 (11%)
Total in hospital, 1 January	243	426	423	418	514	676

On 31 December 1911 there were 699 in the asylum: 114 mentally handicapped (16 age under 15), 61 epileptics, 21 brain-damaged (7 with GPI), 33 with senile dementia, 381 with a psychosis.

TABLE 9.4
Admissions and discharges, 1935–81

	1935	1939	1943	1947	1951	1961	1971	1981
No. admitted	199	243	249	278	279	903	811	526[1]
No. discharged	81	177	164	202	178	828	799	492
No. who died	81	59	74	91	66	75	100	41
Total in hospital	766	792	740	732	744	795	560	(350?)

1. There were 359 admissions to psychiatric wards at High Wycombe and Milton Keynes; these people might otherwise have come to St John's.
The available beds increased after 1947 and 1951. After 1971 a separate Department of Mental Health of the Elderly took patients aged 65 and over elsewhere, reducing St John's figures for admissions and deaths.

from unobserved fits and suffocation among the epileptics that the asylum was modified to allow for the proper care of such a number of special sufferers.

Table 9.4 gives figures for 1935 and, like those to 1911, they reflect a long period of little change, although later years show an increase in admissions annually without any increases in beds as Dr Skottowe's policy of out-patient clinics, community care, and encouragement of willing patients took effect. The rise in admissions was matched by a rise in discharges, and from 1961 the number of people coming in, staying a short while, and going home again becomes enormous, output almost equalling input, and the latter up to four times what it had been in 1935. Finally, in 1981 the use of the hospital declined as new centres of treatment opened and the over 65s were taken into a separate department, as the mentally handicapped had been in the 1930s.

A look at the annual deaths in Tables 9.3 and 9.4 shows it represents a roughly steady proportion of all the patients, but if we look only at deaths in the year of admission – that is, mostly of people admitted to die – we can see that in 1881 they reached 18% of the admissions, though more usually they ran about 10%. They must have represented an important part of the nursing and medical work, but of course we do not know how well or poorly it was carried out, compared with the facilities in general hospitals elsewhere. Examination of some of the causes of death, and what happened in 1914–18, is discussed below.

Patients were admitted, some died, some were transferred to other institutions, some stayed the rest of their lives and, quite contrary to popular belief about asylums, a considerable number were discharged home. In a few cases the patients were allowed home though no better than when they came in; in rather more they were markedly improved ('relieved') and a significant number were in fact 'recovered'. Table 9.5 considers only these last in a number of sample years from 1871 to 1941 and shows that the vast majority of the recovered did so within a year of admission, many of them within the half year. Based on the total admission for the year, over 40% of all admitted patients went home again within 12 months in 1871, but the figure was around 30% in most of the other years in the sample. They

TABLE 9.5
Time spent in hospital to recovery

Time spent in hospital	Number of patients discharged in:						
	1871	1881	1891	1901	1911	1935	1941
Less than 1 month	2	2	0	3	2	8	16
1–3 months	13	11	17	10	14	27	55
3–6 months	6	8	14	11	21	17	51
6–12 months	11	5	11	10	22	32	51
Over 1 year	8	2	3	4	11		
Total recovered	40	28	45	38	70	84	173
Total admissions	78	96	157	112	198	199	
% recovery up to 1 year	41%	27%	27%	30%	30%		

Some incompletely recovered ('relieved') people were also discharged. They are included among the discharged in Table 9.3 but not here.

probably represent manic–depressives who got better spontaneously (there was no drug treatment for this group till nearly 1960), and it is interesting how similar the discharge picture is over the years. Possibly with more available doctors and nurses the recovery rate might have been greater or quicker (or at least recovery noticed sooner). Nevertheless, that 30% of those admitted went home is a tribute to some effectiveness of the institution. At the time, however, official statements repeatedly emphasised the ever-growing burden of incurables (and the need for more or bigger institutions) and glossed over the numbers of the 'cured'. Thus on 31 December 1881, according to the annual report, there were "434 inpatients, probably curable 15". This was poor public relations and engendered the myth of the asylum as an eternal prison.

Two cases

As a life story sometimes conveys more than statistics, here are two patients (taken from the case book) who died in 1902 of conditions now curable, illustrating the nursing work demanded, and in the second case a success story.

Case 1

A married chairmaker aged 32 had an epileptic fit for the first time in his life when he was 31, and thereafter over the next year was rather strange in manner. He developed false ideas of his own wealth and importance, and his memory became less good. A week before coming into hospital, just before New Year, he became very restless and excited, and could not be stopped from walking out into the country in the dark at 4 a.m. He talked in a rambling, disconnected manner. Physically he was well nourished, but rather feeble and unsteady. He was admitted on 4 January 1890. The doctor noticed the pupils of his eyes were not equal in size, and did not react normally when a light was shone on them; his speech was unclear and there were tremors of his tongue and facial muscles.

In hospital he was for a while much the same. After eight months he had another epileptic fit, and his speech seemed thicker and more indistinct, and soon thereafter he became incontinent of urine, and sometimes needed catheterisation. He was no longer restless, but he was very simple and lacking in memory. By the end of the year he hardly spoke, and he began to lose weight. He no longer controlled his bowels. After 15 months in the asylum he was no longer walking, but still able to sit up, though getting more feeble and helpless. He no longer took notice of his surroundings, and could only accept small quantities of fluid foods. He gradually slipped into a coma and died on 1 April 1902.

This illness (GPI) was said to be responsible for 10–20% of the admissions in big city asylums, whereas in 19th-century Bucks two to four cases a year were the rule. By 1901 it was suspected, but not fully proved, to be due to a delayed effect of syphilitic infection contracted 10–20 years earlier. There was then no treatment, but after 1917 a cure was found, and nowadays large doses of penicillin are effective, and the illness has vanished from our hospitals.

Case 2

Martha H was a married woman of 24, a lacemaker and by religion a Dissenter, and had twice been in Hanwell asylum before her marriage. On 15 March 1853 she was admitted to the asylum as she had been ill since the birth of a child two weeks earlier. She was very excited, raving at the top of her voice, spitting at those around her and tearing her clothes. She had religious delusions, wanted to throw herself out of the window, was violent to the nurses, and smeared her room all over with faeces. Nine days later she was well, and she went home the following month.

Four years later, seven days after another childbirth, she was back in the asylum, noisy, violent, scratching and trying to bite the nurses, tearing her clothes and bedding. Her case notes report that she said that "Our Saviour was in constant communication with her, telling her she would not die but that He would take her to heaven that day. She threatened to take her husband's life, having a mission from Our Saviour to do so." By two weeks she was very much improved in every respect, but three weeks after that she suddenly became excited again, laughing and crying and saying she saw beautiful visions. She was secluded, but in three days was completely well again. Three weeks after, she went home, with a financial allowance.

Another four years later, in 1861, she had another breakdown, not after childbirth this time, but again excited, raving, attempting to bite and scratch.

> "She tells me she has a great work to do for Jesus Christ, that she has been with him during the night and that he has so changed her that she can look at the sun with impunity and walk without shoes or stockings without feeling the road. She has perfect control over the Devil and often converses with him to cheat him! She was very thin, and would not eat, and was given broth and arrowroot."

In two weeks she was much better: she made lace and attended the chapel. Just over two weeks later she again had a brief episode of excitement, then recovered and went home again.

Nine years on (January 1871, now aged 42) she began wandering about the village at 4 a.m., knocking on doors, singing hymns and psalms, and almost nude because she did not want clothes and the Devil was soon coming to take them all away. Again she recovered after a week in the asylum.

In 1873 she had two short attacks, and again in 1880 and in 1881, when she said she was in labour to bring forth the Brazen Serpent; she shouted fire and murder and tore out her own hair to swallow it; as before, quick recoveries. There were further attacks, notably 1896, 1901 and finally she was admitted again 23 August 1902, with incessant laughing, talking and singing, continually dressing and undressing, very thin and undernourished. From 10 October she was confined to bed with bronchitis and cardiac failure and died a month later aged 72.

This recurrent mania would today have been treated, with lithium carbonate or haloperidol for instance, and would almost certainly have been prevented after the first or second attack – thus sparing her about 15 admissions to hospital, and quite possibly prolonging her life.

Only a minority of 'cured' patients returned after initial discharge (see Tables 5.2, p. 62, and 9.3, p. 120). To return so many times, through a whole lifetime, was distinctly uncommon.

Some causes of death and World War I

A primary function of any hospital is to save life. We cannot know how effective or futile the asylum was in this regard, though there can be little doubt from the lack of staff, the lack of training and experience of the staff, and a few anecdotes, that avoidable deaths occurred. It was only after the coming of the National Health Service that a psychiatric patient had a good hope of getting specialist medical or surgical advice, nursing and treatment (and then, not invariably). But one can look at the published annual statistics of survival in hospital, and at the ages and duration of stay of those finally dying.

A small number admitted every year stayed a long while (Tables 9.6, 9.7). Of those dying in 1918 alone (a year of high deaths) 24 had been 20 or more years in hospital, 4 had been over 30 while 14 had been 20–24 years – almost three per year persisting thus. Taking 1917 and 1918 together there were 10 patients (five of each sex) who had been over 30 years continuously in the

TABLE 9.6
Survival in hospital

Years	No. admitted	No. remaining in asylum	
		after 10 years	after 20 years
1860	85	12	7
1865	84	18	9
1870	108	11	3
1875	139	13	8
1880	91	10	1
1885	85	9	6
1890	96	10	?
1895	138	11	?

asylum, the two patients who had stayed the longest being aged 55 and 56 years. Clearly, some people could survive in the asylum and live to old age there.

And yet, because of overcrowding, poor sanitation, and other factors such as inadequate nursing, some diseases were endemic. An admitted patient in good health was threatened at times by dysentery and gastroenteritis, by influenza and pneumonia, by epilepsy, and above all by tuberculosis. Every year tuberculosis claimed deaths, and every year for an extremely long time the Committee refused to do anything about it – to provide the known sufferers with isolation from the rest who had not yet caught it, and the treatment (fresh air and food) known to promote the healing of the lungs, or the laboratory facilities (many simple) to aid in early diagnosis and progress. Of course the requisite knowledge was not available in 1853 – it was by 1900 or 1910, but it was not fully utilised at Stone till after World War II, 40 and more years on.

Tables 9.8 and 9.9 show the annual deaths for 1868 and 1910–26 with some causes. Dysentery and influenza *deaths* imply many more cases who survived, with good nursing and medical care of the time. GPI was a disease known to kill, usually in two to four years from diagnosis, and simply gives a baseline of steady death determined by the number of new cases admitted year by year. Senility means merely that the patients were old. The deaths from tuberculosis were judged by the annual inspectors as about twice the number to be expected in an asylum of this size.

TABLE 9.7
Length of stay of the 503 patients in the asylum on 31 December 1900

Length of stay	No. of patients
Less than 5 years	233
5–10 years	94
10–20 years	82
20–30 years	56
Over 30 years	33

126 *Eighty years of nursing*

TABLE 9.8
Causes of death in 1868

	Males	Females	Total
Cerebral or spinal disease			
apoplexy and paralysis	0	1	1
epilepsy and convulsions	2	2	4
general paresis (GPI)	2	1	3
maniacal and melancholic exhaustion	1	1	2
inflammation, and other diseases of the brain, softening &c.	2	2	4
Thoracic disease			
inflammation of the lungs, pleurae and bronchi	4	0	4
pulmonary consumption	1	0	1
disease of the heart, &c.	2	1	3
Abdominal disease			
inflammation of the stomach, intestines, or peritoneum	0	0	0
dysentery and diarrhoea	1	2	3
ovarian dropsy	0	1	1
Exanthemata	0	0	0
Erysipelas	0	0	0
Cancer	0	1	1
Anaemia	0	0	0
General debility and old age	0	5	5
Accidents	0	0	0
Suicide	0	0	0
Total	15	17	32

Average age at death: males 49, females 66. Taken from the asylum's annual report.

The revealing thing in Table 9.9 is to look first at total deaths. In the first quinquennium (1910–14) it lies between 61 and 77 per year (average 67), and in 1923–26 between 59 and 77 (average 68). But in each of the war years, 1915–18, it rises to attain the startling figure of 257, one-third of the patients in the asylum. It drops to 138 in 1919, and thereafter in the peace years is at something like its pre-war level.

The same thing happens to tubercular deaths, too high already in 1910–14 (there should have been none), doubling and trebling with the war, to reach 65 in 1918 alone, and dropping back again in peace. The international influenza epidemic of 1918 arrived in the autumn (when 291 patients and 51 staff caught it), with 22 patient deaths resulting in that year. Obviously this was not the cause of the majority of deaths. Table 9.10 shows that the deaths were not confined to the elderly, but included adolescents and children. Nor were they to be ascribed to a sudden rush into hospital of already physically ill people.

The Board of Control noted such increased deaths (though not necessarily on such a high scale) in other asylums and made some inconclusive studies of the phenomenon. Many superintendents thought it was due to malnutrition, but the Board was content to ascribe it to the war. There is little doubt that the Bucks Committee had cut the patients' rations to below survival level in an attempt to save money, and were responsible

TABLE 9.9

Numbers of deaths and some causes, 1910–18

	1910	1911	1912	1913	1914	1915	1916	1917	1918	1919	1920	1921	1922	1923	1924	1925	1926
Total asylum population, 1 January	622	676	699	695	682	701	820	788	763	677	623	720	737	609	675	670	707
Total no. of deaths	62	77	61	67	67	81	110	129	257	138	71	90	92	59	77	63	58
from tuberculosis	4	12	11	10	8	14	28	19	65	24	6	5	16	7	8	6	7
from GPI	10	8	5	5	3	6	8	8	7	7	1	9	5	3	6	3	6
from senility	8	4	10	7	7	15	16	32	42	36	19	28	28	16	15	12	18
from influenza	1	–	–	–	–	–	–	1	22	6	1	–	3	–	9	1	–
from dysentery	3	2	2	2	1	2	2	–	2	–	–	–	–	–	–	–	–

TABLE 9.10
Wartime deaths, by age

	20–39	40–59	60–79	over 79
		Age group		
All patients dying after at least six months in hospital				
1915	10	13	19	7
1916	15	25	30	6
1917	16	32	31	9
1918	52	69	52	11
Patients dying within six months				
1915	6	6	9	6
1916	6	11	9	5
1917	6	9	12	11
1918	16	21	20	3

Note that deaths among recently admitted patients (within six months) rose only in 1918, while deaths among those in hospital for over six months rose every year, and were distributed across all age groups.

for over 300 extra deaths. As soon as the dietary was improved (albeit at considerable cost) in 1919, the death rate dropped. Thereafter food was never a problem.

Eventually in the 1950s and 1960s it was possible to eliminate tuberculosis and the other endemic infections from the hospital. With drugs, epilepsy and GPI ceased to be common or to require hospital admission, and manic–depressive illnesses were usually controllable. New specialisms appeared – in the mental health of the elderly, in rehabilitation of chronic psychotic sufferers – and new professions to take over part of the investigation and treatment of patients. Since 1936 in Bucks the focus of activity had been shifting gradually from the mental hospital into the community, with day centres, and professionals calling at home on sufferers. The purpose for which the asylum was built in 1851 and which it was able to take on about 100 years later, was by then largely satisfied by other means.

A building which was nearly always ill-adapted to the uses for which it was put, out of date, and insanitary until relatively recently, can now be dispensed with. The charm of the original building, the grounds, the distant view, are not sufficient reasons for carrying on in the old ways. Back in 1850 the Lunacy Commission believed in small units and tried to persuade magistrates not to build giant institutions for 1000 or 2000 patients, but they were unsuccessful. Now we are going back to small units, to a humane scale, but no doubt they will bring their own problems.

IV. Treating illness

10 Revolution

When Dr Skottowe arrived in April 1935 he took over a hospital which was backward, run down, ossified, still living in the 19th century. Dr Kerr had served it for 38 years, overlapping by 12 years with Humphry's half century. Long runs of work like this in one place in a professionally isolated environment were not conducive to up-to-date practice or facing up to chronic problems. Neither Humphry nor Kerr had been able to guide the Committee in its priorities: they were of course only employees, and in Humphry's case at least regarded as of somewhat inferior social status.

The hospital was overcrowded, understaffed, the Superintendent had only one doctor to assist him (with 700 patients!), tuberculosis and dysentery were endemic, and the medical care was out of date. Social work had failed to take root in 1923, occupational therapy likewise in 1932. The ideas and values of both had been put forward but not grasped, and so the necessary space and staff not allocated. As for the buildings, the greater part were about 80 years old and never planned to accommodate so many people. The separation of patients into groups requiring different types of care (called 'classification') – the physically sick, the epileptic, children, the elderly, the new acute admissions, the convalescent preparing for discharge – was not possible because of the size and layout of the wards. There was insufficient space, too, for resident nurses, who in any case expected better facilities (bathrooms, common rooms, bedsitting rooms) than their 19th-century predecessors.

The report of the Royal Commission of 1926 and the Mental Treatment Act 1930 had proposed out-patient clinics, a hospital laboratory, an occupation officer, but none of this was happening in Bucks. Of course it was by no means the only mental hospital stagnating in this way.

A turn in public opinion

The 1926 report is such a landmark in the history of British psychiatry that some account of it needs to be given. It was to be Dr Skottowe's guide in the many changes he made, and its influence continued through the later Acts of 1959 and 1983. It began by analysing the then state of the law governed notably by the Lunacy (Consolidation) Act 1890, and the current ways of dealing with "persons of unsound mind". The asylums or mental hospitals dealt with only a fraction of such persons. It was perfectly in order for people with mental illness of any kind to be kept and perhaps treated at home.

But if the family wanted such a person 'put away', most often because he was a danger to himself or others, or a severe nuisance, then he had to be certified before he could be sent to a public mental hospital or compelled to enter a private institution. For a private patient a relative got statements from two independent doctors (certificates) giving the mental abnormalities observed in the patient, and then petitioned a magistrate to order him to hospital, for which the family would pay.

For the patient and family without sufficient means the relieving officer or overseer of the poor (or sometimes a policeman) had first to be convinced that the patient could be considered a pauper, and then he arranged to take the patient directly to a magistrate, or first to a workhouse, and to get a doctor's certificate in support. In all cases it was the magistrate who decided whether to order the hospital to take him in. Discharge could take place only if the relative asked to have a patient back from private care, or the visiting committee of the asylum or governors of the workhouse discharged the pauper. Of course doctors could advise about this, and their advice was often taken.

The doctors who certified for admission were not specialists but general practitioners who knew very little about psychiatry or how to examine for psychological symptoms and signs. In consequence a "person of unsound mind" usually had very obvious abnormalities, as might be evident only after a long period of gradual development. Certified patients were not likely to be the early cases who might be the most curable. The division into private patient and pauper which had seemed appropriate in Victorian times had become an over-simple class distinction. The non-paying patient could well be a respectable citizen with a regular job and small means, and to be admitted to a public hospital he had to undergo a sort of conversion to pauperism and possibly pass through a workhouse.

The asylums had begun as places to put people whose relations were all dead, or who were found wandering and unidentifiable, or who were dangerous to others. Gradually they became more acceptable to the public as places where mad relatives might go to be treated, or to be looked after if they needed more prolonged care. The general attitude tended to be one of compassion. This seems later to have been replaced to an extent by fear and disgust. The Lunacy (Consolidation) Act 1890 was based on the idea that the mad and the sane were quite distinct, and that society must exclude the mad, hold them apart and shut them away, possibly for ever because a person who could not maintain a normal social equilibrium could not be trusted.

The important thing was to guard against mistakes of diagnosis. The law went into considerable detail to avoid depriving of liberty someone who might not be mad; but once the decision was taken it was not easy to be regarded as sane and set free. The asylum became less an institution of care or cure, more a prison. No doubt the medical superintendents who year after year in their annual reports emphasised the ever-increasing burden of incurable inmates contributed to this pessimism. They made it easy to overlook the fact that 30% of each year's new admissions to hospital actually got better and went home again, many in less than six months. The emphasis was on locking up for life.

The Royal Commissioners of 1926 were mostly lawyers and Members of Parliament, but two of them were medical men. None were psychiatrists or related professionals. They took a new look at lunacy, rejecting the 1890 Act. They affirmed there was no clear demarcation between mental illness and physical illness. Mental illness might show a derangement of conduct in many different ways, only a few of which were dangerous or a severe nuisance. It was often accompanied by physical symptoms also, though these could be greatly overshadowed by the mental. In some cases mental illness was undoubtedly caused by physical agents (brain injury, alcohol, syphilis); and physical illness quite often had accompanying psychological symptoms.

Because there was no difference of substance between so-called mental and so-called physical illness, or between mild mental illness treated at home and severe illness compelling admission to an asylum, the time had come to put the emphasis on diagnosis and treatment of all illnesses without artificial distinctions. Instead of excluding a fraction of patients from society, all should be offered treatment, and the law should ensure that everyone received proper treatment and was protected against neglect or cruelty. The law should infringe individual liberty only for as long as the patient's symptoms needed this for his or her own or the public safety. Certification should be a last resort, not the first step to get into hospital. In fact the mentally ill should be treated in general hospitals as well as mental hospitals, and anyone who wanted admission into either should be free to enter without legal involvement as a voluntary (later, informal) patient. Discharge would become a purely medical decision. In addition local authorities should establish out-patient clinics where those not needing hospital amenities could be seen. In this way early and mild cases of all kinds would receive help.

The Commission went into the details of hospital care, taking wide evidence from a variety of experts and others. They said no mental hospital should have more than 1000 beds, and that a medical superintendent could not hope to govern well anything bigger, even if relieved of what was often a crushing burden of general administration. No asylum doctor could honestly care for more than 200–250 long-stay cases or more than 50 new acute cases at once. Also doctors needed to be taught psychiatry, and given time to learn it (in the 1920s the London County Council gave its staff three months' study leave in rotation to gain post-graduate training).

These maximum case loads and the need for study leave meant that mental-hospital staffs would have to be much larger. Nurses needed more training, and increasing their numbers led to recruitment of mature women as well as girls, and flexible posting so that they nursed both sexes, in contrast to the rigid division between males and females enforced in the Victorian asylum. The evidence the Commissioners had suggested was that one nurse to ten patients was about right, though a ward of disturbed cases might require one nurse on duty to four patients, after allowing for those away on leave or undertaking other duties.

The Commissioners also commented on hospital food. In many places nothing was offered after a light tea around 5.30 p.m. until breakfast at 8.00 a.m. This was inadequate. It also appeared that some institutions only allowed 5 s per week per head for food (1926 prices) which they thought bound to be insufficient. They wanted every patient to have his or her own towel, toothbrush and supply of toilet paper, and an end to such practices as having to share bath water with two or three others.

Why was there this great change of opinion? Undoubtedly World War I had quite a lot to do with it. This was a time when brain injury and alcohol were seen to cause mental problems, and the Army to be faced not only with soldiers suffering from psychoses but otherwise from shell-shock, hysterical paralyses, and disorderly action of the heart (anxiety state) which were psychological in cause and treatment. This created public sympathy, and soldiers who had to enter mental hospital were treated as private patients at the Government's expense. The work of Freud and Jung and their followers was becoming known. Malaria had been used successfully to cure general paralysis of the insane (GPI) while barbiturate drugs could give beneficial sleep and prevent epileptic fits, helping to a new feeling of therapeutic optimism. Revelations of the brutalities of asylum life also played a part, such as the account of his wartime locum in Prestwich asylum by Dr Montagu Lomax in his book *The Experiences of an Asylum Doctor*, published in 1923, which provoked a public inquiry.

Skottowe's vision

With Dr Skottowe's arrival the hospital's annual reports changed dramatically. It doubled in size, to 48 pages, because he used it to explain the statistics, discuss the aims of the work, and to educate the county councillors. Innovations and future projects, with costs, were described with such enthusiasm that it was sometimes hard to distinguish achievement from hope. But the reader was invited to think what the hospital was for and how it should develop. He was lucky to have a Chairman, Mr Darvill, prepared to be enthused and supportive.

In his first report he told the Committee and the councillors generally that they were not simply running an asylum but were responsible for providing a mental health service for the whole county. This meant there had to be co-ordination with other council services, and in September 1935 the Visiting Committee held a conference with representatives of the Public Assistance Committee (responsible for workhouses) and the Mental Deficiency Committee (responsible for care of the mentally handicapped) to consider whether anything further could be done for the senile, the harmless chronic psychotic, and the mentally handicapped adults admitted to the asylum. Skottowe's survey suggested that 191 patients did not need mental hospital care, and that if senile patients continued to arrive as they had been doing the already overcrowded building would soon need over 300 more beds. This ground had been gone over before, but never by round-table discussion strengthened by actual statistics. It did not lead to any relief for the mental hospital (the workhouses were already holding on to some of their mentally ill), but later next year, in July 1936, at a suggestion from the Board of Control, Skottowe was appointed as consultant to the five workhouses in the county, which allowed him to see patients there before they were certified and sent to the mental hospital, and also to educate the masters of those places in the handling of difficult people and what mental treatment could and could not do. In the years 1939–43 he was seeing about 70 new cases a year in this way.

Another crucial innovative step was when in August 1936 he got the Committee to agree that he and other senior doctors could visit urgent or difficult cases at home at the request of general practitioners (GPs). This carried no fee other than travelling expenses, but it allowed him to educate the GP, fending off some admissions by teaching home management, explaining the value of voluntary admission in place of certification, and assessing patients who were house-bound or could not attend a clinic.

In line with the Mental Treatment Act 1930, a psychiatric out-patient clinic was opened in September 1936 at the Royal Buckinghamshire Hospital (Aylesbury's then general hospital), and Skottowe was made an honorary consultant to the hospital in January 1937, and allowed eight beds in the medical wards for the use of psychiatric patients. The out-patient clinic prospered: 98 new cases in 1941, 182 in 1942, 276 in 1943. Of the 276 in 1943, only six had been in contact with the mental hospital before, and 32 were referred from the medical and surgical services of the hospital; another 22 were servicemen. GPs had referred the majority (189), and 146 were subsequently treated at home by the GP with clinic advice. Only 38 out of the 276 went on to mental hospital; a further nine were treated as in-patients in the Royal Bucks Hospital. The clinic expanded to two days a week, and was run by two junior and two senior doctors from the mental hospital.

Here was evidence that there was much mental illness in the community which would never have come into the asylum, and that the medical and surgical patients of a general hospital could sometimes benefit from psychiatric advice. Where such in-patients were seen in the ward it was called a pastoral visit, and such visits were quickly extended to other hospitals in the county and carried out by other members of Skottowe's staff. The numbers of patients seen in the wards like this in 1951, Skottowe's last year in post, were: Royal Bucks, 52; Tindal (Aylesbury), 13; Stoke Mandeville, 111; Amersham General, 25; Wycombe, 38. Some of these patients were people who had attempted suicide and needed physical revival before psychiatric assessment. Others developed mental illness after surgery or after childbirth, both known potential causes, and yet others were difficult diagnostic problems, a tangle of physical and psychological pathology.

The success of the Royal Bucks clinic encouraged the foundation of others. A fortnightly clinic was opened at King Edward VII Hospital at Windsor in the south of the county, with Dr P. Holliday from Stone and Dr Henry Wilson as consultant from London. It was 35 miles from Stone, and with the coming of the National Health Service (NHS) the whole area was transferred to the care of St Bernard's Hospital at Southall in the North West Metropolitan Region. Aylesbury is only three miles from Stone, while Amersham and Wycombe are about 17, half the distance to Windsor. Clinics were eventually opened in Wycombe (1952), and in Amersham (1953), and in Bletchley in the north of the county (1957). For a time, from June 1949, there was also an out-patient clinic at Stone, at the mental hospital itself, especially for urgent cases. In 1950, when 366 new cases were seen at the Royal Bucks Hospital, another 84 attended at Stone, and the total attendances at the two clinics came to about 2000.

This development of a county mental health service reached its administrative apogee when Skottowe was made County Psychiatrist in October 1947, consultant to all hospitals and homes run by the County Council. The reorganisation at the inception of the NHS took all the hospitals away from the County Council and produced quite a new administrative pattern. Nevertheless the mental health service created in 1935–48 continued to develop along the same lines and proved enduring for the succeeding 40 years.

Staff for the work

Such a dispersed community service required doctors. Yet up to the end of 1934 the County Council had employed only Dr Kerr and his assistant Dr Anthony, and had turned down proposals for more, in spite of the Board of Control's repeated criticism that this was totally inadequate for 600 in-patients and an annual intake of about 150 new cases. It was fortunate that Dr Kerr's sudden death and Dr Anthony's serious illness had precipitated a crisis.

When Professor Shaw Bolton agreed to act as Locum Superintendent he made it a condition that two experienced psychiatrists must be appointed to support him, and Dr S. R. Tattersall and Dr Edith Booth (Mrs Tattersall) were selected: they were to be the backbone of the staff for the next quarter century.

As far as Dr Skottowe was concerned this was only a beginning. His first step, in 1935, was to get Committee approval for the appointment of unpaid clinical assistants. Dr Margaret Carter was the first of a long line of these, doctors who were willing to work for a time without a salary, for the interest of the work and to gain extra experience. The following year the Committee agreed a new staff structure. Dr Tattersall became a permanent senior assistant medical officer (at £600 p.a.) and two new posts of resident junior assistant medical officer established (at £350 p.a.). Dr Joan E. Greener, with public health experience, and Dr J. Sawle Thomas, previously working in general hospital psychiatric clinics, were appointed and sent to learn neurology as clinical clerks at the National Hospital for Nervous Diseases at Queen Square in London for three months.

With World War II, clinical assistants were called for military service, and no further doctors were available. Dr Skottowe took advantage of the evacuation of the Middlesex Hospital Medical School from London to Aylesbury to persuade one of their psychiatrists, Dr Spencer Patterson, to join him and to offer teaching to senior medical students and get them to put in time helping in the hospital. Staff expansion had to wait for the end of the war.

Teaching was a part of Dr Skottowe's enthusiasm for clinical work, and led him to hold regular case conferences. To make time for this he tried where possible to delegate administrative work. The visiting Committee met monthly in peacetime and every second month in wartime and had four subcommittees: estate and farm, finance and contracts, general purposes, and special purposes (later, housing and catering). Matron, chief male nurse, engineer reported directly to the main committee, and the farm bailiff, the clerk and steward, or other appropriate officer to one of the subcommittees. Skottowe did not go to the subcommittees, or play a big part at the main committee; he expected to keep in touch informally, but let departmental heads act at meetings.

An example of Skottowe's ability to make good use out of lucky chances came very early after his arrival. In January 1935 the Mental Hospitals Association and the Mental Hospital Workers Union had agreed between them that indoor workers (i.e. nurses) should drop their working week from 59 ¾ hours to 54. To do this meant either that staff would do more overtime to cover the work, or that the numbers employed would have to be increased. He got the Committee to accept the national agreement and to expand the staff to an extent which would have astonished his predecessors. The increase was far more than simply to compensate for the shorter working week – 16 extra men and 18 extra women, plus 6 extra domestic staff. The cost of this was to raise the weekly maintenance charge per patient from 18 s 6 d to 21 s, or by over 12%, a jump which the Committee seems to have taken in its stride. Enough men were recruited to start the 54-hour week on the male side by September 1935. The women took to February 1936. The church estate purchased in 1934 had included the old vicarage, which was now turned into temporary accommodation for the new staff.

By 1938 the nursing staff had been further raised to a total of 60 men and 65 women, the best it was to be for a very long time. It appeared sufficient for the work, which with the introduction of physical treatments made greater demands on nursing knowledge and skill. But World War II took 20 men away to the Services, and the women began to leave too, for better-paid (and more obviously patriotic) work in armaments factories. This loss of staff, occurring on a country-wide scale, induced the government in 1941 to pass the Mental Nurses (Employment and Offences) Order, which said that nurses working in mental hospitals under nationally agreed wages and terms of service could not leave their jobs except with the employer's consent.

By 1942 male nurses had dropped to 35 and female to 46. By day the nurse : patient ratio was 1 : 15.5 for men and 1 : 17.2 for women (compare this with the Royal Commission's recommendation of 1 : 10); by night the ratio was six times worse – there was hardly any night supervision. Unfortunately once the war was over it proved extremely difficult to recruit nursing staff, especially women. At the end of 1947 there were still only 49 men and 46 women, and it looked as if the hospital might have to close its doors for lack of staff.

The nursing shortage created by the war meant inevitably a curtailment of treatment. Early in 1939 Mr Snookes, a charge nurse, had been sent to the North Riding Mental Hospital to learn about occupational therapy. When he came back he was to instruct the male staff in this aspect of treatment, but the war intervened. Insulin coma treatment, then regarded as a valuable treatment for schizophrenia, had to be given up in 1941 and was not resumed till 1952, shortly before the new antipsychotic drugs came in and made it seem redundant.

Progress in treatment

From the beginning Dr Skottowe introduced new and effective treatments. Patients with GPI were offered the malarial fever treatment which killed the *Spirochaetes* of syphilis which were responsible, acting over many years, for the developing mental illness, and stopped it in its tracks. Patients with pernicious anaemia (a known rare cause of mental illness) were cured with injections of liver extract, eventually discovered to contain cyanocobalamin, vitamin B12, as the active agent. Barbiturates were used to control epileptic fits, and to provide sleep treatment (continuous narcosis) for many cases of anxiety and excitement: psychotherapy was used in the calm end-stage of this treatment. All these methods had been developed from 1920 onwards.

When in 1936 insulin shock treatment for schizophrenia was announced in Vienna it aroused enormous international interest and the Board of Control sent Dr Isabel Wilson to study it and report back. Dr Skottowe saw a demonstration of it in Edinburgh, and then Dr Sawle Thomas from Stone was given a travel grant to spend his leave in Vienna in 1937, and in the following year began the treatment in Bucks. The idea was to induce unconsciousness in a controlled way by lowering the amount of sugar circulating in the blood by an insulin injection. Once the patient was in coma he or she was quickly revived again with large injections of glucose, and food by mouth. This was done every morning of a five-day week, for as many as 40 times. It required skilled nursing and constant medical attention, and had dangers (particularly when there was delay in ending the coma), but the results seemed impressive. A nursing sister trained in medicine as well as psychiatry was appointed in 1939 to oversee the insulin ward, to supervise all medical treatment on both sides of the hospital, and to act as a nursing tutor.

Electroconvulsive therapy (ECT), the production of a series of controlled epileptic fits by electrical stimulation, had been discovered in 1938, but was viewed at first at Stone with a certain scepticism. However in 1942 the first machine for delivering the controlled stimulation was purchased (for £68-7-9) and because of its effectiveness, it was soon to become the main treatment of serious depressive illness. It continued to be of great therapeutic importance for the next 30 years, and is so even today.

Pre-frontal leucotomy, a brain operation in which certain nerve fibre connections to the frontal areas of the brain are cut, had been introduced by the Portuguese doctor Egas Moniz in 1936, and was greatly publicised by Drs Freeman and Watts in the USA in 1942. It could produce amazingly good results in abolishing chronic intractable depression, or ending excitement and violent disturbance in some schizophrenics. It could also produce amazingly bad results, but in the absence of other effective therapy for long-term cases its exploratory use seemed justified. From 1950 for a year or two Professor Sir Hugh Cairns and his neurosurgical team from his University department at the Radcliffe Infirmary, Oxford, came regularly to Stone, making use of the new operating theatre, opened in 1945. Psychological assessments were made by May Davidson of the Warneford Hospital, since there was then no psychologist at Stone. When the new drug era opened with the arrival of chlorpromazine (Largactil or Thorazine) in 1953, leucotomy fell very much into the background and the neurosurgical link ended. In a much modified and improved form, with few bad effects, this kind of operation is still available at a few centres in Britain as the treatment of last resort in severe chronic intractable depressive illness.

The operating theatre, which had cost £1000, was there primarily for the use of the honorary consultant general surgeon, Mr R. H. Gardiner, appointed in 1941. His work was mainly the repair of hernias, and the excision of benign tumours and other routine operations. Before 1945 the patients had to be transferred for a short while for surgery to the general hospital, which feared the mad and insisted on a psychiatric nurse accompanying each patient – a very expensive use of staff. With the training of two male nurses as theatre assistants the mental hospital needed only a visiting anaesthetist and the surgeon to cope with its own surgical cases. The drawback was that there were not a great many of them in the year, and so the staff had rather little experience either in theatre or in pre- and post-operative nursing. With the growth of pastoral visits and out-patient clinics at general hospitals, and the spread of psychiatric teaching, the general hospitals became less nervous about psychiatric patients and began to accept them like ordinary patients. This gave them better nursing and treatment post-operatively, and saved specialists' travelling time: the Stone operating theatre became redundant less than ten years after it was opened.

The pace of this acceptance nationally was very variable. I recall a London teaching hospital regularly accepting surgical cases from a large mental hospital in 1954, yet less than 50 miles away and 14 years later I was approached by one senior surgeon to remove to a mental hospital one of his in-patients who had become mentally confused. This was an old man of 70 who needed a prostatectomy to let his urine flow freely; he had come into hospital for operation three days earlier, but had become confused about where he was, as sometimes happens with the elderly. The surgeon refused to operate, or keep him, so I telephoned another general hospital 20 miles away who took him and operated.

The period from 1939 onward was one of increasing collaboration by local specialists in medicine, surgery and pathology, helped by the wartime Emergency Medical Service and by the evacuation of the Middlesex Hospital students and teachers to Aylesbury. They were useful allies above all in dealing with tuberculosis and gastrointestinal infections, where a laboratory plays a big part in diagnosis. Attempts to get a small laboratory built and staffed at Stone got nowhere, and the hospital began to pay £200 a year for the services of a private laboratory in London. Then Dr Skottowe managed to convert a storeroom with the help of some old furniture, got Dr Ilse Hertz, the wife of Dr Hertz, then his clinical assistant, both refugees from Frankfurt, to act as a laboratory worker (until they emigrated to the USA) and persuaded the Committee to pay for equipment and chemicals.

Dysentery and enteric fever should be stamped out, said the Board of Control visitors in 1937, when 18 fresh cases of dysentery had just appeared, possibly linked to defects in the sewage system, which was to be renewed in 1940. The previous year there had been a panic over a case of typhoid diagnosed only post-mortem, and patients and staff had been offered anti-typhoid immunisation. Gastroenteritis, with a few deaths each time, kept appearing, in spite of attempts to prevent it. Two severe epidemics occurred in 1943. That in January, affecting 61 patients, was apparently not an infection but due to a heat-resistant poison that had got into the milk (probably from bacterial contamination). After laboratory investigation it resulted in greater care for cleanliness in food handling. That in July was bacillary dysentery, however, spread by a carrier in the kitchen (someone with the bacteria, but not made ill by them). First 48 men were affected, then 28 women, with one death. It was impracticable to do bacteriological tests on all the contacts and therefore all patients, whether ill or not, were given a six-day course of the antibacterial drug sulphaguanidine, and the epidemic was killed.

In January and February 1945 dysentery attacked 81 men and 132 women, plus five male staff, but there were no deaths. While the poor washing facilities and old inadequate drains and the lack of nurses continued, stamping out the infection seemed impossible.

Tuberculosis also continued to be a problem: there were twice as many cases as in other asylums of comparable size. No doubt the overcrowding contributed to this, but gaining control depended on chest X-rays and laboratory sputum examinations, and being able to isolate sufferers at an early stage before they could spread the infection to others. Healing was encouraged by good food and fresh air. In 1936 the doors from ward 16 into the garden were widened so that beds could be pushed through into the open (weather and staff numbers permitting), so that 21 of the 45 bed-bound patients could benefit. In 1941 the county architect created temporary verandahs for this and three other wards at a cost of £600, which gave shelter from the elements, but separate isolation chalets had to wait till the NHS came in. By then there were drugs like streptomycin, isonicotinic acid hydrazide, and para-aminosalicylic acid to strike at the infecting bacteria.

Overcrowding! Building? Improvisation

Except for the decade 1904–14, the hospital had been overflowing with patients, especially women, for most of its existence. By 1935, with 773 patients in residence, it had gone beyond overcrowding in the sense that it had been forced to park 20 chronic female patients in Bodmin (Cornwall), and another 20 plus 20 men at Littlemore, Oxford, at an annual cost of nearly £3550. However, this bill could be set against the just over £4000 brought in by 50 private patients then at Stone. Of course the need for extra buildings had been raised in 1912 by the visiting Commissioners in Lunacy, but World War I had provided a reason to stop the planning. The Board of Control, successors to the Commissioners, had begun to raise the matter of new buildings again in 1925, and frequently thereafter. The Committee fought the matter off with various excuses, until in 1929 they finally began to develop plans. Dr Kerr's sudden death in 1934 provided another opportunity to call a halt.

When he arrived, Dr Skottowe attacked the building problem with great vigour. He wrote a short history of what had happened since 1912, and he started measurements and careful calculations to work out the present true capacity of the buildings, and the rates of admission and discharge of patients then and projected as likely in the next ten years. His predecessor had not thought it necessary to go into such details. Skottowe's full report was printed for wide distribution as a 50-page booklet by the Committee. He used the Board of Control's 1933 statement on the amount of space each patient needed: 40 square feet by day and 50 by night. On this basis the existing building should accommodate 345 men (in 1935 actually 355) and 359 women (in 1935 actually 418); therefore the hospital had 69 too many patients on 31 December. Add the 50 patients parked elsewhere and this meant 119 extra beds were needed to satisfy present commitment. But patients were still accumulating at an average 16 a year. These figures were for total numbers of patients, but patients were of very different kinds with very different needs: the senile and the young for instance.

Since 1912 the proposal had been to build a separate block for the new patients, to keep them away from the chronically and the recurrently disturbed. Skottowe looked at the new admissions of the previous five years. If each of them had had to stay up to six months in a special unit it would have required 70 beds to be self-contained. Similarly a villa of 50 beds for convalescent patients was needed, and he proposed two further villas of the same size for the overflow chronic patients, with modifications in the main building to suit the actual numbers of sick, etc., being encountered. It was characteristic of his plans throughout to use the arithmetic of Bucks rather than national averages from Board of Control reports. Having laid out the work he estimated how many resident and non-resident nurses were needed to do it. To attract staff and house them, a separate nurses' home was required, for 73 but capable of expansion, with its own kitchen and a restaurant to hold 200 (for non-residents as well).

The Committee accepted these ideas and asked the county architect to prepare plans. They would have to be approved by the Board of Control as suitable, and then by the Finance Committee of the County Council who would have to find the money. But first there was a difficult issue to settle: what would be the best way to provide the central heating, hot water and power for the laundry and kitchens that the new buildings totalling perhaps 300 people would require? A new boilerhouse and new engineering workshops were envisaged. There were additional plans to build the matron a bungalow, and for the clerk and steward a house. This last was able to go straight ahead, and "Holmesdale", built by Cannon, Green & Co. of Aylesbury for £1425, was nearly ready by the end of 1936.

To scrap the boilers of the old building and to have one modern heating and hot-water system for all buildings, new and old, as the Committee had wanted to do in 1914 would have cost £4000 more than any other solution. A compromise, to leave the old building, in future to house only 609 patients, with the old heating, but have a new system for the new buildings, was agreed by the Board of Control, and there began to be hopes that building might start in early 1939. The estimate was it would cost £110 000. But in May 1938 the County Council announced it would not find this money, or indeed anything for 1939, but could offer only £20 000 for 1940/41. Dr Skottowe hastily prepared a memorandum explaining the urgent need for more accommodation for patients, and declared that the admission hospital and the nurses' home would suffice for the present. The Council replied in July that they could not find additional money. This was reported to the Board of Control who in August wrote a stern letter to the Council saying they appeared to be in breach of their legally imposed duty to provide for the mentally ill of Buckinghamshire. The implication was they might be liable to prosecution if they persisted in their policy.

This threat in August led the Finance Committee of the Council in November to refer the matter to their capital expenditure subcommittee, who eventually found some money to proceed. August 1939 brought World War II and justified a stop to the project. Dr Skottowe was not beaten yet. He pointed out that the population of Bucks was now rapidly enlarging with evacuees from London. This would increase the calls on the hospital's services. There was also the possibility they might have to take patients transferred from elsewhere, as had happened in 1914–18, although in the event this did not happen. He therefore asked for just two open villas for 85 patients. No special engineering would be needed, they could be built for £15 520 plus £2500 for furnishings and £500 to make an access road. The Board of Control approved, but the County Council said no.

In 1944 he had another try. By then there was a good deal of experience with pre-fabricated huts for barracks and hospitals for the Emergency Medical Service (EMS). He asked if he could have two EMS huts to hold 30 patients each. The Board of Control thought it over and said "no, only one hut" (presumably afraid that the more huts they sanctioned the less permanent high-class accommodation would ever be built). The Committee was incensed by the reply and decided to insist on two huts anyway. There were wartime controls on all building, so they needed official approval, however. Eventually it was agreed that two huts could be put up, with the proviso that they must be erected by hospital staff and patients and not by outside labour. This was at a time when many staff were away on war service, and it effectively slowed down the construction. It had been hoped that the two huts would be ready as an admission unit by the end of 1947, three years after the original proposal, but the male ward opened only in October 1949, and the female ward not till after April 1950 – though the delay at the end was caused by a shortage of nurses. By then the NHS was in operation, and the new hut wards were named after the secretary and chairman of the former visiting committee of county councillors, "Crouch" and "Darvill" wards (Fig. 10.1).

The permanent admission hospital so long sought was not built till after Dr Skottowe had left. Called "Beacon House" and providing for 32 women and 28 men it opened on 20 June 1959. This was 20 years after the outbreak of war had interrupted advanced plans, and 31 years since the Committee

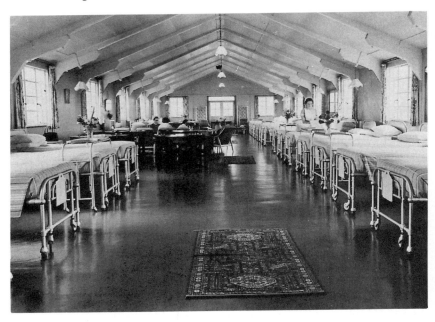

Fig. 10.1 Darvill Ward in 1950 – an Emergency Medical Service hut

had agreed to it; 47 years since it was first proposed. It was built by the NHS: the County Council had managed to dodge the cost after all. Ironically, it was to be closed as an admission unit about 20 years later.

So far, Dr Skottowe had met only with defeat on overcrowding. The end of the war gave him another idea, a way of gaining extra space without going through the traumas and delays of building plans, finance and rejecting committees. Special buildings were expensive to create, and were difficult or impossible to sell if they became unnecessary. Buying existing houses in the village could be a very different matter. "Peveril Court", originally an Edwardian country house just outside Stone, behind the Buglehorn Inn at the Hartwell corner of the main road, had been bought in 1939 by a London insurance company, and they had evacuated their offices to it, and put up long huts in the grounds to house their staff. The Committee purchased the house, huts and 19 acres of land in November 1945, as soon as the insurance company moved out. Nominally it was to create an early-treatment or neurosis centre, but in fact this never happened, and Peveril provided chiefly a nurses' home, with seniors in the house, juniors in the huts. In addition some of the huts were later removed to the hospital and became homes for the nurse training school, for the ECT treatment unit, for occupational therapy in 1948, and for the offices for social workers in 1945. Later, two other big houses were bought: "Stonecroft" on the main road near the village centre in July 1949, and St John's Lodge on the southern outskirts

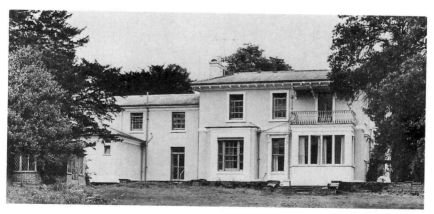

Fig. 10.2 St John's Lodge, purchased in 1953 as a male nurses' home

of the village at the end of 1953, the latter as a male nurses' home (Fig. 10.2).

The necessary refurbishment of the Peveril huts still required Board of Control approval. General plans were submitted to them in January 1946, detailed plans on 16 March, and they sent back provisional approval on 23 April. The work was at once put out to tender. Full approval from the Board of Control followed on 4 September, and the Ministry of Health issued timber permits on 7 November. Meanwhile suddenly in October the Board proposed totally new plans for converting the huts. The Committee was understandably annoyed and refused to discuss the matter. The Board then yielded and refurbishment began. But the Board got something of its own back in another matter. During 1946 the Committee bought motor transport: a 22-seater ex-RAF coach to carry nurses back and forth to Peveril, a lorry for farming the 19 acres there, a coal lorry, and a light pick-up truck. They engaged driver-handymen, and planned a garage to keep the vehicles in (Fig. 10.3). The Board had to approve the plan, and received it in September 1946, but by March 1947 they had still not replied, and so no garage had been built. It seems an absurdity of central bureaucracy that the Board of Control, a body to promote the humane care and treatment of the mentally sick, should have been controlling the building of a garage or the refurbishment of a temporary staff hut somewhere in the English countryside.

All these big houses served a turn in housing staff, including doctors and domestics, but ultimately they all had to be disposed of again. They helped the hospital keep running, but whether it would have made better financial sense to put up new buildings for the staff instead of patching up old ones is open to discussion. The lack of a proper nurses' home was certainly one factor in the inability to recruit women staff. In some small ways the nurse's life eventually improved. A central canteen, a six-bay pre-fabricated hut, was opened in 1946, so that no nurse need any longer take her meals on

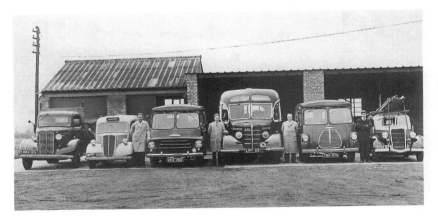

Fig. 10.3 The hospital's motor transport

the ward, and mealtimes became a real break in the day. Dr Skottowe encouraged the formation of staff social and sports clubs and relaxed the Victorian segregation of the sexes off duty.

Improvements

The big building plans of 1939 had included a new laundry. When the overall plan was blocked because of the war, Mr G. W. Harrison, chief laundries officer to the Surrey County Council, was brought in to advise, and a £6000 scheme of laundry reorganisation was approved by the Bucks County Council in November 1939. It was turned down by the Board of Control in 1940 but the Committee declared they would go ahead all the same and it was finally completed in 1942.

Earlier, other improvements had been under way. The hospital was rewired and two 100 kW electric generators installed. Seven and a half acres of land to the south of the hospital were bought in 1937 and used for a new sewage disposal plant jointly with Aylesbury Rural District Council, opened in July 1940. In 1937 the six staff cottages just across the main road from the hospital entrance were given bathrooms, and next to them an additional five pairs of cottages were built. Electric lighting was provided from the hospital generators. Six of these new houses were used temporarily to house 29 female nurses.

Less expensive improvements could be made directly by the Committee without prior County Council approval. Some of them had often been proposed by visitors from the Lunacy Commission or the Board of Control but ignored by previous committees, for example fitting surgical wash-basins and hot and cold water in the infirmary wards, and giving wards 9, 10, 11, 12 sanitary annexes with extra toilets and basins (at a cost of only £100, so not much can have been done). Ward 9 was given a garden. Clinical rooms were established in the main wards so that patients could be interviewed and treated in privacy. For the staff, equipment for the nurses' lecture room, nurses' dining-room, and cycle sheds were some of the changes of 1935 and 1936. The hospital got an internal telephone and fire-alarm system for £395, and reception of BBC radio programmes throughout the building for just under £100-worth of GEC equipment.

Reports of the inspectors over many years referred to the kindly handling of the patients, the absence of complaints from them when interviewed in private, and their good relations with the staff. Whatever the other medical and nursing deficiencies, the suggestion was that the patients received humane care. Under Dr Skottowe standards of care began to rise. Seclusion was less used than in Dr Kerr's time, six of the 18 wards were unlocked, and an average of 9% of the patients (75 or so) enjoyed 'parole', which meant they had freedom to come and go through the day. Sports were encouraged, patients' football and cricket clubs with regular matches, bowls, quoits, sometimes athletics; and a sports pavilion was built. He had early reclaimed the recreation grounds 'stolen' by the farm. (However they were ploughed up again during World War II.) Groups of patients went on picnics and coach tours, and regular cinema and social events were held in the hospital.

In spite of the overcrowding the annual admission rate increased, largely with voluntary patients, but the increase was balanced by shorter stays and an increase in discharges. Annual admissions increased by 50% between 1935 and 1949 while the total number of in-patients on 31 December fell slightly each year: 792 in 1939, to 719 in 1947. Thus admissions in 1934 were 175 (20% voluntary); in 1938 about 240 (56% voluntary); in 1947 278 (63% voluntary). This was only achieved by vetting the proposed admissions and trying to limit them to those who needed treatment which could only be given in hospital (e.g. ECT) or who had to be removed from home to save a fraught situation, where the patient's disturbance threatened the peace of mind if not the property of the family.

Previously admission had sometimes been for kindly storage – the elderly, the mentally handicapped, the chronically disabled of one kind or another, who were inoffensive and simply needed ordinary care. Now through good telephone and personal contact with GPs and workhouse masters, and the out-patient clinics, patients could be diagnosed and treated without admission, or if admitted could soon be discharged before they were cured, because their treatment could be continued at a clinic. A waiting-list for admission was established. It is obvious that the work the hospital was undertaking was quite different in 1936–46 from what it had been in 1900–34.

The war

In 1914–18 the asylum had been forced to take an excessive number of patients to free space elsewhere for nursing the military wounded. This did not happen in 1939–45, but the Buckinghamshire population greatly expanded as people were evacuated from London, and some of them proved to need psychiatric treatment. The hospital itself was in a rural area, away from military and industrial targets of great importance, and was therefore not required to do much in the way of air-raid precautions. In 1938, 22 artisan staff were trained as a fire-fighting squad, six on duty each day, and a gas decontamination team was established in the laundry. When gas masks were issued, 360 patients refused to wear them; roughly two-thirds of the men but less than half the women accepted them. It was therefore planned that a number of rooms should be gas-proofed, and 165 windows covered with removable gas-tight wooden shutters, but the Home Office discouraged this and it was not proceeded with. A combined military and civil disaster exercise held in 1942 showed that every member of staff would have to be on duty at once to cope with patients and damage. Fortunately the hospital in fact was never attacked, and came through the war dilapidated but unscathed.

In contrast also with the earlier war, the food situation remained good, thanks to the notably successful national rationing policies of the Ministry of Food. In-patient deaths did not rise, there were no epidemics of influenza and respiratory infections, and deaths from tuberculosis varied from year to year as they had previously done without showing any increase. Dr Skottowe had a detailed scientific assessment of the dietary made in 1943. It seemed the patients should be getting on average about 2684 calories per day, with 61 g fat and 77 g protein (a sedentary *worker* was officially recommended a little more than this). There was a possible deficiency of vitamin C, so he arranged for the farm to plant 120 each of blackcurrant and gooseberry bushes, 50 apple trees, 500 raspberry canes and 1000 strawberries (supplemented in 1945) to provide for patients in future years. In fact all was well.

Nutrition did not suffer in spite of the staff shortage. The cook retired in 1944, her deputy was away at the war, it was impossible to get a trained catering officer, and of the six women who undertook the total burden of the kitchen only two were regular staff. Loss of staff was the biggest problem created by the war. The engineer lost three men, stores, bakery and general office two each; the farm lost one. Twenty male nurses, nearly one-third of the whole staff, went off to the war, and there was a fear that a further 26 would be called. However, this time the Government created reserved occupations (farming, nursing) to ensure important civilian services were not denuded. There were losses too on the women's side: the female nurses had dropped to 11 too few by 1940, and recruitment of women became a problem.

Reconstruction

With the return of peace in 1945 came staff changes. In December Mr R. W. Ward took over from Mr E. J. Jeffries, who had seen 31 years, through both world wars, as clerk and steward. Mr C. H. Mulcuck became head male nurse, chosen from 41 service (and 120 civilian) candidates. During the war, notably in 1943, social work with out-patients had been helped by Miss Findlay, regional representative of the provisional National Council for Mental Health, when the local authorities failed to provide – another example of Dr Skottowe's ability to take advantage of lucky circumstances, in this case Miss Findlay's presence in Aylesbury. But in September 1945 the hospital acquired a full-time trained psychiatric social worker of its own in the person of Miss K. M. Benger. The medical staff now had five full-time doctors and was talking of the need for six or seven. But the big problem was nurses, particularly women. In May 1946 there were only 18 nurses on duty by day (for part of the day only 14) on eight wards with 400 patients. Some staff were working 128 hours per fortnight (the official 54-hour week gave 108). The official Rushcliffe report was recommending a 96-hour fortnight.

Not a single recruit was obtained from an extensive advertising campaign or from repeated appeals to the Ministry of Labour, and the hospital was approaching a crisis. It had long been the case that it could not staff itself with local people and needed recruits from the north-east of England, Wales and Ireland, and they had to be offered good accommodation and facilities. Five new nurses appeared in July, and later one or two more from Ireland, and it was eventually possible to start the Rushcliffe scheme. Most hospitals ran this as a series of eight-hour shifts, with two days off per week; the Bucks staff preferred 12-hour days at this time, with a block of five days off in the fortnight, perhaps because it allowed those from far away to get home occasionally.

In 1947 the General Nursing Council approved the hospital as a complete training school for mental nurses, on condition that resident accommodation was provided for men away from the wards and they were given their own bathrooms (where one was then being shared between six), that the sluices in the infirmary were modernised and hot water laid on for all patients' hand-basins. The Committee decided to honour these obligations.

The National Health Service took the hospital away from County Council control in July 1948; the whole basis of finance and management changed. Although Dr Skottowe stayed on as Physician–Superintendent (significantly his title had been changed from Medical Superintendent in 1944 to emphasise that he was a clinician), till early 1951 his creative contribution was over. He had lost most of the battles to renovate and extend the buildings and relieve the overcrowding. A nurses' home remained a dream and the staff had shrunk to crisis point. But he had created a true community service, with out-patient clinics, visits to general hospitals (and beds in one of them), and domiciliary calls. It was a new way of working, with the mental hospital open to the public and taking many more patients, mostly for very short stays.

When he left it was to become Consultant Physician at the Warneford Hospital, Oxford, without any of the burdens of finance, recruitment, or committees to distract him from the care of patients. He continued as before to write medical articles, and when he retired he played a big part in starting up the Wessex Postgraduate Medical Centre near Southampton, providing systematic psychiatric teaching.

Notes

The background to the setting up of the Royal Commission of 1926 and where some of its ideas came from is given by:

HARDING, T. W. (1990) "Not worth powder and shot": a reappraisal of Montagu Lomax's contribution to mental health reform. *British Journal of Psychiatry*, **156**, 180–187.

The *Report of the Royal Commission on Lunacy and Mental Disorders* was published by His Majesty's Stationery Office (cmd 2700, 1926).

11 Breakthrough?

The year 1931 had marked a revolution for the mentally ill. Henceforth the medical services were to provide for all of them and not just the mad, the lunatics; and furthermore, treatment not social exclusion or isolation was to be the aim. It was a complete change in ideology.

The year 1948 brought a second revolution, the start of the National Health Service (NHS), which for the mental hospital meant a complete change in organisation. All the local finance was swept away. Henceforth all the money would come from the Treasury in Whitehall, channelled through the Ministry of Health to the Regional Hospital Board at Oxford. The Board would decide how much of the year's block grant for hospitals would be spent on mental health services, and within that what would go to each of the various mental hospitals now within their jurisdiction (the former county asylums of Berkshire, Northamptonshire, Oxfordshire and Buckinghamshire, the Warneford Hospital, Borocourt Mental Handicap Hospital, and others). Dependence on local finance was finished. There was an end to control by county councillors, weighing up how much of the rates to spend on education, roads, and social services, in competition with mental illness for limited funds. That system had repeatedly led to excessive parsimony and mistaken policies by the elected politicians of the County Council, people who could be totally ignorant of the facts of mental illness, and sometimes unsympathetic to the sufferers, yet given the power to determine their fate.

In the new organisation nobody was elected by popular vote. Members of the Regional Board, and locally of the Hospital Management Committee (HMC), which partly took the place of the previous Committee of Visitors, were all selected by the Ministry of Health from people with some interest in the hospital services and often representing a particular expertise. Thus a general practitioner, a pharmacist, a trade unionist, someone from the local university, a businessman, a clergyman, and so on might be invited to serve for a fixed period and without payment, meeting weekly or monthly on a policy committee or subcommittee. But in addition the Board had a paid staff of professionals – architects, engineers, doctors, nurses, accountants – to act daily as advisers and administrators. This organisation was a recognition that hospitals are complex machines, that there is a whole technology to be mastered for a successful medical or surgical service, and that the amateurism of the county council, like its money, was inadequate.

The Board's specialists were interested in promoting good practice and knew what was going on in other regions. They consulted with specialist groups of senior doctors from their own region. The Psychological Medicine Subcommittee at its regular meetings brought together psychiatrists from the different mental hospitals, who benefited by meeting their colleagues as well as the Board's staff face to face. They were no longer isolated, each in his county organisation, and could be sure of a sympathetic discussion of their work problems with an appropriate specialist. They were not subservient to their HMC because they were employed by the Regional Board and not by their local committee. But the HMC remained the employer of the rest of the staff, and a first control on expenditure.

In addition to money and professionalism, the NHS brought improved staffing and training. The Royal Commission of 1926 had preached that psychiatric hospitals were in principle no different from other hospitals, and there was no dividing line between mental and physical illness. Now the NHS brought all hospitals together in one organisation with the same design and rules for all. If a general hospital was staffed with junior doctors in training (senior house officers, registrars) and permanent seniors (senior hospital medical officers, consultants) then a psychiatric hospital should have them too – at once a step to a bigger medical staff in the mental hospital, to better training, to the promise of a professional career in the service, and to better recruitment. If the general hospital employed medical auxiliaries such as laboratory and X-ray technicians, physiotherapists, almoners and other specialists, then in principle so should a mental hospital. Since the researches of the last 75 years had revealed more and more cases of mental illness with an important physical component, the psychiatrist might need the help of diagnostic tests and machines quite as much as the general physician. The NHS made it easier to upgrade the quality of medical and nursing practice in the psychiatric setting.

The narrow outlook of a county council, intent only on its own parochial affairs, within its county boundaries, was replaced by a broader, more national outlook.

The NHS was to be a way of spreading knowledge and good practice nationally as well as making it available to all citizens equally – there were to be no private patients in NHS psychiatric hospitals. It had been recognised in the years leading up to 1939 that neither the voluntary hospitals (royal infirmaries and the like) nor the county and municipal hospitals could be adequately financed by charity, charges or the local rates: only the state possessed the necessary millions to pay for the special equipment and teams of trained people required for modern medicine in all its branches. This, and experience of the wartime efficiency of national organisation in food rationing, in evacuation of children, and in the Emergency Medical Service, helped to bring the NHS to birth.

The birth of St John's

After the war Dr Skottowe seemed to have lost some of his drive and creativity. Of course the impending reorganisation (the NHS was to start in 1949) put a blight on plans and spending money. When the NHS came, it removed South Bucks (the Beaconsfield, Gerrards Cross, Slough area) from the hospital's catchment area, and this should have eased the work by 60 new in-patients annually, but this made no difference to the admission rate in practice. In the next 20 years Bucks was to be the fastest growing county in Britain as people flooded in from London to Bletchley and the new town of Milton Keynes, to Aylesbury and High Wycombe and to Amersham. The extension to Amersham of the underground railway from London, the opening of the M1 motorway, and the spread of light industries, encouraged expansion.

Dr Skottowe stayed for five years after the war to see the new organisation in and the Aylesbury Hospitals Group Management Committee get to grips with things. One of their first acts was to change the hospital's name to try to remove the stigma of the title 'mental hospital', and after considering several options (such as 'Hartwell') they settled for St John's, because it was built on the glebe land of Stone Parish Church of St John. But they had responsibility for several local hospitals – the Royal Bucks, Tindal, Manor House (and after 1950 also took over Stoke Mandeville, which was both a spinal injuries centre and a general hospital) – and became preoccupied with the many problems general medicine and surgery were presenting. Their then Chairman, Captain L. M. Paterson, a business man from the Bifurcated Rivet Co., was also soon one of the 18 members of the Regional Board. He was joined there by Skottowe in 1951, when he removed to Oxford, which may not have been a help to his successors. Dr A. A. Petre was Locum Superintendent for a few months. Then Dr S. L. Last arrived.

Last was a very different personality from Skottowe and the two did not get on. Skottowe was outgoing and sociable, a good talker and a bit of a showman, ready to negotiate informally over a drink in the bar, a piano player, a bridge player, a car rally driver. He supported and enthused his staff, so that the hospital laundress was glad to clean his clothes personally and a senior doctor colleague to service his Rolls Royce regularly.

Last on the other hand was reserved, dispassionate, cautious and self-critical, not a man for the pub and easy warmth. In consequence he had to struggle for improvements, rely on logical argument and apposite questioning, where Skottowe might have won more easily. He was horrified by the state in which Skottowe had left the hospital, the kitchens crawling with cockroaches, the ward sanitation medieval, the overcrowding, the endemic tuberculosis and dysentery. He had come from one of the newest and most modern hospitals in Britain, Runwell in Essex, opened in the mid-1930s. He had been there about 14 years, latterly as deputy superintendent, and was noted as a pioneer of clinical electroencephalography: he had a research department for this specialty at Runwell as well as his routine clinical work, and also attended one day a week as an assistant at the London Hospital in Whitechapel. Originally of Austrian nationality he was an MD (having studied in Berlin) and had been an academic neurologist in Bonn before coming to Britain in 1934 at the age of 32. Here he had re-qualified and worked as a psychiatrist at Whitchurch, in Cardiff, and at St Crispin's, in Northampton, before Runwell.

He was determined to improve the condition of the in-patients, not only with proper hygiene and civilised domestic amenities and comfort (Fig. 11.1), but with less rigid discipline all round, more humanity, more talking with patients and listening to their complaints. He did not want patients kept in bed for two or three weeks as a measure of control, he did not want out-of-date drugs such as sulphonal (a hypnotic) used. The staff were inclined to resent what they thought of as a lack of leadership and support (after Skottowe's bravura and discipline). One of them

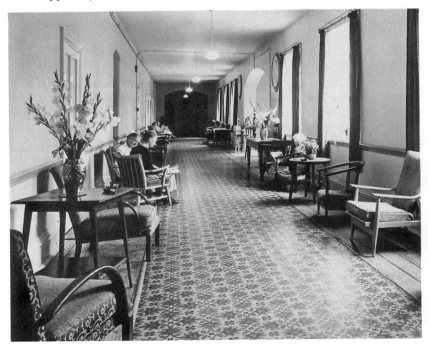

Fig. 11.1. A long gallery in the old building as a day room, 1962

complained when Last was investigating how a patient's jaw came to be broken, "you are always on the side of the patients," which was in fact where he thought he ought to be.

His, and the Committee's, initial failure to function successfully emerged pointedly in 1953 over the matter of building the new admission wards for which Skottowe had fought so hard in the 1930s and '40s, and which were so much needed to reduce the chronic overcrowding. In the September the Ministry of Health gave the Regional Board an extra £1 million, and the Board decided to spend about a seventh of it in the mental health field. New admission wards would be built at two psychiatric hospitals (Littlemore at Oxford and Fairmile near Reading), while a third (St Crispin's, Northampton) would get two new villas for women in-patients. There was nothing for St John's. The HMC protested vigorously and was told "we thought you wanted a nurses' home" (which they most urgently did: many nurses were still living in rooms on the wards amid the patients). In the end St John's got its admission wards (Beacon House), but not until 1959, after the first stage of the nurses' home in 1955.

The Board in fact became well enough disposed to St John's to spend enough money to make up for many past deficiencies. In Last's ten years as Superintendent there was a great deal of building, enough to do for the rest of the hospital's existence. Beacon House (60 beds) with furnishings cost over £150 000. Sanitary annexes, a proper provision for the first time in the old building of enough showers, wash-basins, toilets and baths, cost about £70 000. A modern big nurses' home was erected on land to the north of the main road in 1955 and 1962), together with more semidetached houses for married staff (including doctors). Chalets to isolate the tuberculous were put up in the grounds, and by 1956 the old enemy was finally defeated. In 1957 there was a new laboratory and a new preliminary training school for nurses. In 1962 a new boiler-house for the whole site and an industrial workshop for 200 patients opened, while a big house in Aylesbury (Byron House) was converted at a cost of £8000 to be the first day hospital. Figures 11.2 and 11.3 show what St John's had become. Thousands had to be spent on the big houses acquired in the village, particularly St John's Lodge at Stone (acquired with hesitation in November 1953, with dry rot and leaking water mains). They were white elephants, wasteful of money, but for a time necessary because of the delays in providing new buildings. St John's Lodge became a male nurses' home.

During Last's early days there were plenty of minor improvements also, new bed-linen, the hospital rewired throughout, and electric light provided for the first time in the chapel, which also received a second-hand organ from the Buckingham Road Methodist Church in Aylesbury. There was a new fire-alarm system, a new car park, and electric tea urns for the wards, an important patient amenity. A patients' shop and cafe was built in 1957 near the chapel, with a loan of £7000 from the Regional Board, repaid from the shop profits afterwards.

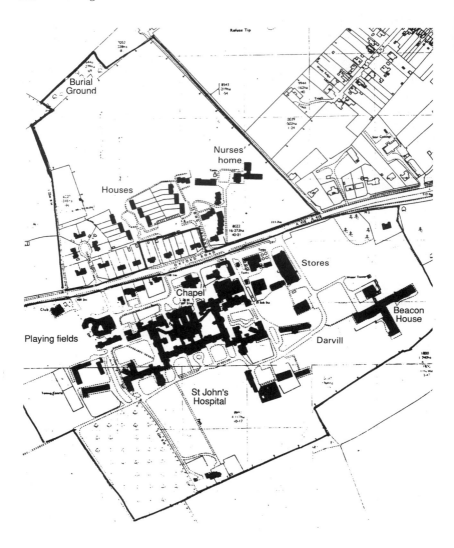

Fig. 11.2. Plan of the hospital in 1975. Compare this with Figs 3.3 (pp. 36–37) and 5.3 (p. 69)

All these advances demanded endless committee work, and Last resolved to try to change his Committee. He asked them all to declare their particular interests and only one mentioned mental health. He drew attention to the fact that Stoke Mandeville Hospital by itself was a major part of the Committee's financial concern and left insufficient time and interest for St John's. The Board, recognising this, established a separate St John's and

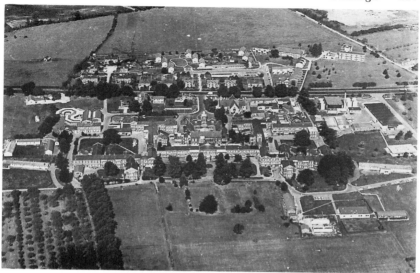

Fig. 11.3. An aerial view from the south of the hospital. At the back, across the road, are the staff houses, with the nurses' home at the extreme back right. This side of the road on the right is the new boiler-house, with stores and Darvill Ward a long horizontal block. In the foreground on the right is the nurses' training hut

Manor House HMC from 1954, with Mrs K. White, a politically experienced former mayor of Aylesbury, as the new and concerned Chairman, and Dr Last got on well with her. When in 1957 the overcrowding had reached 15% he persuaded her to hold a monthly HMC meeting at the hospital at 7 p.m. instead of 11 a.m., so that Committee members could see what 15% actually meant at night. Mrs White found it a searing experience. The upshot was the loan of a ward of 25 beds at Stoke Mandeville to house chronic patients until Beacon House could open – not enough, but something.

The enormous backlog of neglect to be made up, which was not confined to St John's, led the Board in late 1952 to ask the Ministry of Health for more money for psychiatry, after they had tried various stratagems to stem the outflow of money – freezing wages and salaries for a time, forbidding increase in any category of staff without Board approval, and fixing staff establishments. They were told to manage on their annual financial allocation, but the Nuffield Provincial Hospitals Trust began an investigation into hospital costs, a year-long study of 12 hospitals across the country, which included St John's as the only psychiatric hospital. The NHS had no research unit, but relied on two voluntary charities, the King Edward Hospital Fund for London and the Nuffield Provincial Hospitals Trust for the provinces, to study the workings of the NHS and recommend improvements. Hospital statistics were still in a very primitive and often misleading or useless state, and hence decisions based on them had good chance of being wrong. For the

Ministry of Health a hospital's annual costs were totalled (with a certain amount of inspired guess work) and divided by the number of patients treated and the number of days of treatment to express the cost as that of the average in-patient day. This was a meaningless figure because it took no account of the different treatments different patients had, of variations in the size, age, and staffing of a hospital, and so on. The Trust showed it was easy to get a finance department to adopt departmental costing – wards, boiler-house, laundry, kitchens, X-ray department, operating theatres and so on costed separately – so that people could see where the money was going and the effects of small changes in practice. In consequence, as part of the research, the St John's accounts became full, modern, and up to date, helping the administrators to see why they had to spend so much and to predict what might happen if they tried to cut spending here or there.

The Maudsley influence

The staff:patient ratio was not satisfactory when Last arrived, and it added to his initial dismay. However, in September 1951 Miss B. Michel arrived from the Maudsley Hospital (the postgraduate teaching hospital 50 miles away in south London) as the new matron, and the problem was attacked with a new vigour. First, advertisements were placed in suitable French and German newspapers and travelling expenses paid to candidates: this produced 12 women from Europe. Second, and better in the long-term, Miss Michel went ahead with enthusiasm establishing a nursing school with 50 places. This meant working while learning. The key year was 1952, with appointment of a full-time tutor, design of a hospital badge indicating qualification, and the first annual prize-giving in November. The following year there were more applicants for training than there were places. There was also a vigorous recruitment of part-time staff, prepared to work at least nine hours a week. In 1953 out of 102 staff now on the female side of the hospital, 25 were part-time, and 35 were students (the other 15 students worked on the male side). With more hands at work, fewer patients were being kept in bed, there was less bed-wetting, and fewer sedative drugs were needed. For a time things were better, then they deteriorated again (see below, "Where are the nurses?").

In 1952 Dr D. C. Watt arrived from the Maudsley as a new consultant. He came with a particular enthusiasm for teaching and research. His Maudsley connection, and his friendship with Dr Michael Shepherd (later a Maudsley professor of note) who was then in the RAF at Halton and living in Stone, were important in the future development of the hospital. Further Maudsley-trained consultants were appointed in 1961, 1962, 1972, 1985, and 1988. After 1960, for a number of years, the hospital housed some Maudsley overseas postgraduate students, doctors who could travel regularly for teaching in south London but who lived free at St John's, were appointed as clinical assistants, and received regular teaching from Dr Watt. There tended to be about three at any one time, and several of them were promoted to paid jobs on the junior staff. Space was granted for two years to a social scientist, and collaborator of Professor Shepherd's, Dr Sheila Mitchell, as base for a study of the effectiveness of Bucks' child guidance clinics, and some research projects on the hospital patient population were carried out in association with people from the Institute of Psychiatry.

The treatment explosion

In 1951 there were drugs for epilepsy, and barbiturates for insomnia and anxiety. Excitement could be controlled by large doses of barbiturates or with injections of morphine and hyoscine. For depressive illness and some schizophrenia there was electroconvulsive therapy (ECT), for other schizophrenia deep insulin comas, or the brain operation of pre-frontal leucotomy (which sometimes did irreversible damage). Psychological treatments were of minor effectiveness in serious mental illness. Suddenly, one after the other, new ranges of drugs appeared which changed a few aspects of a person's mental state, without adversely affecting many others, including consciousness, which the earlier drugs did. They were drugs which had much more effect on abnormal mental states than on normal everyday thinking, feeling and behaviour, and their psychiatric effects were discovered by accident and quickly applied in clinical practice, in St John's as elsewhere, from 1954 onwards.

Chlorpromazine had first been synthesised as an antihistamine and then found to be of use in anaesthesia. This led to the idea that it might be calming in the restless, overtalkative, overactive manic patient, and it found some symptomatic use here. Then it was tried on excited schizophrenics with good results, and when extended to the non-excited proved of great value in modifying disordered thoughts, abolishing aggressive or morbidly suspicious feelings, and even delusions. There was a rush by chemical laboratories to produce a whole family of drugs with similar effects. Many of them had the same phenothiazine nucleus as chlorpromazine, but with different atoms attached here or there. Others belonged to the chemically dissimilar butyrophenone series – haloperidol, and pimozide. From 1954 chlorpromazine (Largactil) was in clinical use, and the subject of research by Dr Watt both in practical use and in psychological effects – the latter in collaboration with the psychological department of the hospital.

Imipramine, introduced 1957 as a possible substitute for chlorpromazine, was found to be helpful in abolishing quite severe depression. Again a whole family of similar drugs emerged, the tricyclics and tetracyclics, which could be used to abort or shorten both mild and severe depressive illnesses. Hospital stays were shortened, fewer people needed to come into hospital but could be managed as out-patients, and the use of ECT began to decline. The effectiveness of chlorpromazine was such that insulin coma treatment also rapidly declined, and leucotomy was mostly rejected.

The new drugs were valuable in the early treatment of a wide variety of psychiatric illness. Chlorpromazine was found to have dramatic effects also on a proportion of chronic schizophrenics. People who seemed booked for a lifetime of hospital protection and care suddenly lost a good many of their symptoms and disabilities and were ready for normal life in the community again. However, no one who had been several years in hospital could simply go home and get a job successfully. They had to relearn the prices of things, the developments in the machinery of domestic life. They had to rebuild family relationships, and be accepted as more normal people by friends and neighbours. They had to recover their self-confidence, and ability to act on their own without nursing prompting. Methods of rehabilitation working over months involved nurses, occupational and industrial therapists, social workers, psychologists and medical doctors, in helping the patient through successive stages in a planned relearning and re-enabling series of events.

Social workers helped families to see the patient in a new, changed light, and to sort out some of the tangles of relationships. A married patient might find that the healthy spouse had (understandably) taken up with another partner. A man whose wife was pregnant when he came into hospital 20 years before had to learn to accept a strange young woman in his home as his natural daughter; and she had to accept that her father whom she believed dead all her life was in fact there, alive, in this unknown man.

The new drugs helped only some chronic patients, not all, and those helped were sometimes only partially benefited, but perhaps enough to be able to live out of the hospital even though somewhat disabled. That chlorpromazine was not truly curative became very evident when it was stopped, or its daily dose reduced below a certain level, and all the symptoms of the original illness then returned, and the patient had to return to hospital. Patients were rather liable to stop taking their drugs when they seemed to themselves to be well, and had to be constantly urged and directed to continue, and many family doctors, health visitors and others involved in long-term community care took a long time to learn this, and there were at first many unfortunate relapses. It proved a very great advance when in the late 1960s long-acting phenothiazines were produced, notably Moditen and Modecate (fluphenazine decanoate), one intramuscular injection of which would usually last for two to four weeks. In 1968 St John's established Moditen clinics in Aylesbury, High Wycombe and Bletchley, to which out-patients on these injections were required to go at least monthly for repeated injection and general inquiry about their problems of health and life. A nursing sister, in effect the first community psychiatric nurse in Bucks, began to drive round to these clinics and, most importantly, call at the homes of any patients who had failed to keep their clinic appointment to find out why and to make sure they did not miss the due injection which kept their illness at bay.

Growth in the community

The old mental hospital up to 1935 had been isolationist and inward looking, and Dr Skottowe had started a movement outward, with out-patient clinics and visits by psychiatrists to people at home, in general hospitals and other institutions. Dr Last built on these beginnings with out-patient clinics opened August 1952 at High Wycombe (Dr Watt as doctor), Amersham in 1953 and Bletchley in 1961; the Royal Bucks Hospital (Aylesbury clinic) expanded with the addition of a mental handicap clinic run by Dr G. O'Gorman from Borocourt. By 1958 every week there were four half-day sessions at Wycombe, two at Amersham and seven at Royal Bucks (576 new cases that year). When Byron House, the first day hospital in Bucks, opened in 1962 it also offered an out-patient service, in addition to giving its day patients occupation, ECT and brief psychotherapy.

Child guidance had hitherto not been available in Bucks, but clinics began in 1954 with Dr Edith Booth (who had come to St John's in 1935) doing two sessions weekly at Aylesbury and two at High Wycombe, with the help of a psychologist from the Bucks Education Committee, and a social worker loaned by the hospital. In 1956 she was fully established as a consultant, with eight sessions, and a second part-time consultant was added in 1961, a year in which 160 new children were seen.

This growth was outward from the hospital. Already in 1950 the Oxford Regional Hospital Board had grouped its specialists into Area Departments (of anaesthesia, surgery, psychiatry, etc.) rather than labelling them by a particular hospital where they worked. This enabled them to work freely in the region, and brought together doctors with similar interests in discussions of professional matters. The Bucks Department of Psychiatry was largely the senior staff of St John's, and it was logical therefore that the growth in service should come from them.

They contributed to the community in a third way by regarding themselves as responsible for the education of the general public and of other concerned professional groups (teachers, probation officers, family doctors) in questions of mental health. This took the form both of organising special lectures and the like at St John's and of giving up their free time to talk to community groups about aspects of psychiatry. Over 40 such outside lectures were given in 1960, for instance. A study day for probation officers and 'duly authorised officers' (local government social assistants who brought in certified patients from home) was held at the hospital in 1957, and this led to a series of monthly clinical demonstrations and discussions for them. From 1953 every year there were seven to ten monthly evening lectures at the hospital, mostly by outside speakers of note on subjects such as mental reactions to childbirth, the pathology of epilepsy, a survey of mental health in a rural area, to which all local general practitioners (GPs) and hospital doctors were invited. This expanded later to weekend courses for GPs, and to a regular psychiatry and general practice study group run jointly with Dr Handfield-Jones, a

Haddenham GP. It was in 1957 also that the first hospital open day was held, and 295 members of the public had a look round. By then 19 out of the 24 wards had been unlocked, they all had names (Darvill, Crouch, Kimble, Creslow, etc.) instead of numbers, and garden fences had been reduced to normal heights. Four-fifths of the patients were there of their own free will. Eleven years later there was not a single locked door in the hospital, which seemed to work just as well without.

Ten-year report

Since 1952 there had been a full-time pathological laboratory technician, working under the guidance of the Stoke Mandeville laboratory and providing routine blood tests and a sterile-syringe service. Since then also there had been a clinical psychologist (T. G. Crookes) soon with an assistant. He was very active in research in addition to many routine assessments, and consultations outside as well as within the hospital.

Industrial work for patients had started in 1951 with a contract to pack rivets in plastic envelopes for a company connected with Captain Paterson, the Committee Chairman, but really got going from 1958, and in 1962 got a new light, airy factory where 200 could work. Many firms offered work, and an industrial manager was appointed, though general supervision fell to the nursing staff. Patients could learn to get on with fellow workers, keep regular hours, improve their working speeds under benign tolerant conditions in preparation (for some) for full work in the world outside. They were paid small amounts, according to their work, and the surplus profits were put into a patients' benefit fund. Some small groups of in-patients even went to work in local factories, but then they had to pay for hospital board and lodging, insurance and income tax. In 1957, for instance, 12 women were employed in Aylesbury in Moorhouse's Jam Factory. A social club for patients, the Chiltern, held regular evening whist drives with prizes, so there was something to do when they came 'home'; another small step to normality.

When Dr Last in 1961 gave up as Superintendent and became a consultant at the London Hospital in Whitechapel he left a hospital where the effects of chronic neglect had been largely abolished: new admission wards, new nurses' home, the old buildings modernised, clean, hygienic and fairly civilised, furnishings and decoration to a high standard, many doors unlocked. Tuberculosis and dysentery were abolished. The consultant medical staff had been increased from two to five, and the juniors from one to three, and the work accomplished expanded correspondingly. There had been 281 patients admitted in 1951, the year he came, whereas in 1961 there were 720, and the proportion under compulsion had dropped from 26% to 14%. The new out-patient clinics saw 81 new cases at Amersham and 259 new cases at Wycombe in 1961, the six child guidance clinics 119 new cases in 1961 (these clinics did not exist in 1951).

Not everything was rosy. The nursing situation was shaky, and the hospital was as badly overcrowded as ever – 744 in-patients on 31 December 1951, but 785 on the same day in 1961; it had been over 800 in 1959. Nevertheless, much of the groundwork for a first-class service had been laid.

Notes

The incidence of mental illness in Bucks and its management by the asylum in 1931–33 and 1945–47 is analysed in:

SHEPHERD, M. (1957) *A Study of the Major Psychoses in an English County*, Maudsley Monograph No. 3. London: Chapman & Hall.

12 Changes of direction

The Mental Health Act 1959 cancelled many of the legal rules that had governed asylum work hitherto. Admission and discharge were henceforth entirely medical decisions, with no reference to magistrates or committees. Certification ceased ('committal' is an analogous legal procedure in the US). Now people could be compelled into any hospital willing to receive them, by medical order alone, with the agreement of relative or social worker. Being 'put on an order' meant being under the orders of a senior named doctor, the responsible medical officer or RMO, who made all the legal decisions. The patient's status might be changed to informal, or he might be discharged completely, or he might be allowed home or out and about on leave for a period without the compulsion order being cancelled. The RMO decided. The Board of Control disappeared, and its inspections ended, together with all the rules about seclusion, record-keeping and regular medical examinations of each patient. The medical superintendents lost all their legal responsibilities, as the senior hospital doctors individually took over as RMOs for their patients. Consultant responsibility became absolute, as it already was in general hospitals. No one could over-rule them.

So the Ministry of Health proposed the abolition of the medical superintendent, and advised that the psychiatric hospital should be administered in three independent sections, the doctors under a medical director, the nurses under a chief nursing officer, and all the support services (catering, engineering, portering, stores, gardens, etc.) under the hospital secretary. The three chiefs would decide everything by consensus. The chief doctor no longer had control of the nursing staff, he could not ban any treatment of which he disapproved, he could not lead except insofar as the secretary and the nurses were willing and approved.

The last battle Dr Last fought before he left was to try to get his successor made Medical Superintendent, with the old powers. The Hospital Management Committee (HMC) were divided about it, and the Chairman and Secretary went to the Regional Board without Last's knowledge and asked for a medical director to be appointed. So it was as Director that

Dr D. C. Watt took over from Dr Last in mid-1961. As it turned out this change was not handicapping, because Dr Watt commanded considerable respect within the hospital where he had already served nine years as consultant, and he continued to hold that respect with a widening circle of colleagues in the ensuing 24 years. In consequence people were willing to accept his leadership, and to see him represent the hospital to the outside world. Substituting a triumvirate for a leader could have arrested development of the hospital and even promoted stagnation and disintegration. This was seen in some other hospitals where the consultants elected a medical leader, for three years at a time, to act as chief instead of having an appointed medical director. At St John's Dr Watt's personality carried him through.

He was an enthusiastic teacher, with a passion for scientific research, and he made St John's, while still an NHS area psychiatric hospital, into almost the equal of an internationally known university department. It developed research sections and training for post-graduate students, and this intellectual stimulus helped to raise the standards of medical practice in the hospital as a whole. He was a Glasgow graduate who, after a short experience of general practice, had worked in three psychiatric hospitals: Gartnavel in Glasgow; Shenley in St Albans, where he had been influenced by Dr S. T. Hayward's humane practice and belief in patients' freedom; and the Maudsley in London, where his scientific bent had been encouraged by Professor (Sir) Aubrey Lewis.

From his start as Medical Director he was faced with the same problems as his predecessors: getting enough staff, and reducing the overcrowding. The staff problem had, however, grown; it was no use having posts for doctors and nurses if they could not be filled, or only taken by people who soon left, or worse still proved of poor ability but stayed on. The work had become more complex, requiring more knowledge and experience than 20 years earlier, and also the collaboration of different professions – occupational therapists, social workers, psychologists, medical secretaries, laboratory technicians. It was not the same world as Dr Kerr had inhabited, with his single medical assistant and his nurses recruited from farm workers and shoemakers and domestics. All these specialised professionals had to be recruited.

As far as the doctors were concerned, the existence of a teaching and research programme made it attractive to them to come and to stay. But Watt developed two special ways of getting staff. One was that he could offer free accommodation at short notice to any doctor who happened to call and who seemed suitable to be appointed as an unpaid clinical assistant. The stock of housing built up under Dr Last made this possible. The other was to advertise regularly in the Australasian medical press, offering junior training appointments in the hospital to young doctors, married or single, wanting to gain experience. They would be housed, and the HMC would vote them some pay on an individual basis out of any free monies they had at the time. This remained a local arrangement, without needing to change the medical establishment, which would have required the approval (probably after long delays) of the Ministry of Health. It was a good way of expanding the number of doctors to do the work, especially as Aylesbury to London was only an hour by train with a frequent service, which allowed people to attend courses at the Maudsley Hospital or the Tavistock Clinic, while Oxford University was half an hour the other way by car or bus. A steady stream of people resulted.

Occupational therapists came and went rather rapidly, and the posts could often not be filled. The opening of the industrial therapy factory in Dr Last's time compensated to some extent, and by 1968 a quarter of the hospital population was working there. From 1965 for a number of years the Aylesbury College of Further Education provided courses in the hospital in art, music, dressmaking, cookery and dancing.

The overcrowding and the lack of nurses were linked matters and deserve a separate account (below) as major issues. But a turning point was the recognition that the overcrowding was partly due to a flood of old people who could be separately treated in special beds and clinics elsewhere. The development of new psychiatric facilities in other parts of the county, first at High Wycombe, also began to relieve the pressure.

The separation of the old, like the earlier separation of children and the mentally handicapped, and a tendency to separate drug addicts and alcoholics in special units, was a growing movement in psychiatry. Additionally in Bucks the increasing population was spreading across the county and to at least four sizeable towns. It no longer made sense to concentrate all the psychiatric services for in-patients in one centre near Aylesbury. In 1969 the St John's medical staff and ward facilities were divided equally into three so that the north, the centre and the south of the county could be equally served by separate teams, who could move out into their areas. These separations sounded the death knell of the old asylum/ hospital.

Teaching and research

A look at the annual report for 1966 gives an idea of what was going on under this head. Several consultants provided clinical teaching at their weekly ward rounds, and the clinical assistants (three post-graduates from the Maudsley) wrote up and presented cases to Dr Watt. In addition, in alternate weeks, there was a case conference for the whole staff and a journal club meeting to discuss recent scientific papers of importance. Some junior staff attended an anatomy and physiology course and a psychology course at Oxford, two attended for three weeks of neurology there, and others attended weekly tutorials at the Tavistock Clinic in London or the Warneford Hospital in Oxford.

Monthly evening meetings continued for all levels of staff, and some specifically for the general practitioner group. They were mostly talks by eminent visitors, such as: the results of current therapies in chronic schizophrenia (F. Letemendia); use of statistics in planning mental health services (G. C. Tooth); aspects of leucotomy (J. M. Potter); dealing with marriage problems (H. V. Dicks); management and treatment of anxiety states (W. Linford Rees).

Since 1963 the psychiatric hospitals of the Oxford region had together planned some post-graduate teaching. Dr Watt took a leading part and in 1967 became officially Regional Adviser for Postgraduate Education in Psychiatry. Each year three three-day courses of lectures to broaden experience were organised, primarily for juniors, although seniors found them useful to attend. Each had a main theme: subnormality, child psychiatry, psychosomatic medicine, schizophrenia. They were held in a hospital or an Oxford college (e.g. in 1966, "Forensic psychiatry", at St John's; in 1968, "Treatment", at New College Oxford, later published as a book by Blackwells). When the new university department of psychiatry opened in 1969 this teaching naturally came under the wing of the new professor.

A good local library is important for such teaching, and 1966 saw the appointment of a first (part-time) librarian at St John's. The library already had 580 volumes, and took 24 regular journals. In 1966 a further 82 books were purchased, 45 borrowed from other libraries, and 30 photocopies of special articles obtained. This medical library had begun unofficially in the early 1950s when the hospital secretary simply entered the cost of books each year under the heading "stationery", where it passed unnoticed. When it became known to the HMC it was too well established to be challenged, so it was accepted as a department of the hospital.

Some of the research was financed in the same unorthodox way. When a biochemical research laboratory was set up in Beacon House in 1963 by a simple conversion of unused rooms originally envisaged for deep insulin treatment, which had meanwhile become outmoded, there was no provision for a salaried laboratory worker. The hospital secretary remarked that there was officially a vacancy for a pig-farm manager, although no farm any longer existed. So the research technician went down on the payroll as a farmer and no questions were asked.

Again, expensive laboratory equipment costing several thousand pounds was bought with end-of-year residual money. Each April the hospital, like all NHS bodies, started with a budget for the new year. Any allotted money left unspent by the following 31 March simply disappeared back to the Treasury and could not be carried over. In consequence, in each financial year as its end approached there was a scrimmage to spend any money in hand rather than lose it, on anything which could be bought in a few weeks, such as attractive china or extra chairs. In several years some of this money went on science.

Some research can be done without special funding. For example an analysis of all the coroners' records of suicide and hospital records of attempted suicide in Bucks for several years produced some ideas for better prevention. The hospital itself of course had no research money, and the Regional Board only a trifling allocation, so that when it was necessary to employ an extra secretary for a while, or a sociologist, or a psychologist, or even an extra doctor, for example in following up what had happened to patients after discharge, the Mental Health Research Fund (a charity, now the Mental Health Trust), or the Wellcome Trust, or the Medical Research Council, had to be appealed to for funds, which were not easy to obtain.

In the 1966 annual report there are some notes on just-completed researches showing the variety achieved. Dr Watt himself, helped by a special assistant on a financial grant, had made a study of clinical and social factors in the successful resettlement in the community of chronic patients treated with the new drugs, and rehabilitation thereafter. This was to be a recurring theme in his work: later he made ten-year follow-ups of people after a first episode of schizophrenia and a series of studies of such patients treated with a new long-acting drug taken orally, pimozide. Meanwhile, in conjunction with the staff psychologists, he examined the effects of the new drugs on normal mental processes: reserpine on reactive inhibition in 1966.

Dr Birtchnell, a senior registrar, studied the significance of bereavement in childhood for the onset later of psychiatric illness, and with Sheila Zinkin, a psychologist from Oxford, compared the benefits and drawbacks of treating depressed patients with unilateral as opposed to the conventional bilateral electroconvulsive therapy. Dr Bagg, a consultant, and Mr Crookes, senior psychologist, looked at palmar digital sweating in depressed women. Dr Elkes, with Dr Crammer and Dr Watt and the financial help of the Medical Research Council, began an inquiry into the action of imipramine in successful treatment of depressed people, which worked in only a proportion of them: could success be related to metabolic changes undergone by the drug in the body? The drug was shown to undergo a number of chemical alterations in some of the tissues, and to different extents in different individuals. Was some pattern of chemical change needed for a good therapeutic result?

Stage one of this research revealed a hitherto unknown metabolic step. Stage two involved making a complete count of all the substances resulting from the swallowing of imipramine, and this was done with imipramine specially labelled with radioactive carbon which could be recognised and measured everywhere. It was specially made and given by the Radiochemical Centre at Amersham, because of the successful treatment of several members of their staff by St John's.

Before radioactive imipramine could be given to patients it had to be shown to be safe in rats (known in general to metabolise the drug like humans). For this purpose, rats donated by the Physiology Department of Oxford

University were maintained in a rat room in Beacon House. In stage three, a series of depressed patients (about 30) were treated in the usual way with imipramine and about half recovered, while the biochemistry of the drug was examined in all of them. The side-effects of the drug were worse in those people who were slower to change the drug chemically, but otherwise there seemed no metabolic difference between those who recovered and those who did not. Some had much higher concentrations of drug circulating in the blood than others, but there was no relation to recovery. However, two important new facts came out. One was that chlorpromazine (Largactil) interfered with the metabolism of imipramine. If the two drugs were taken together, as sometimes happened, there would be much more unchanged imipramine circulating than would be the case in the same person on the same dose of imipramine alone. The other was that patients with pronounced obsessional symptoms but little depression might be greatly relieved by high doses of the imipramine.

The problem of the elderly

In December 1962 there were 776 occupied beds; a year later there were 745. For the first time the hospital began to shrink, and there was a steady drop annually, by 230 in ten years (546 occupied beds in December 1972). Yet the Bucks population had increased from 295 600 to 426 300 in the same period. The drop began as a consequence of the discharge of long-stay patients after treatment with new drugs and rehabilitation, was helped perhaps by the opening of a psychiatric ward at Wycombe General Hospital in 1967, but was undoubtedly pushed on by a new policy for the treatment of the elderly at the end of the 1960s. This new policy was a response both to the overcrowding and to the shortage of nurses.

There was always a substantial minority of the over-60s among the year's new in-patients in Bucks (see Table 9.3, p. 120: 21.5% in 1861 and 1871; 24% in 1901 and 1911) but it remained a fairly constant fraction until after World War II. In England and Wales as a whole the fraction was smaller (about 12%) but showed a similar post-war rise: 16.1% in 1946, about 20.5% in 1951, with a greater proportional increase in the number of women. In Bucks in 1951 there were 93 admissions of patients aged over 60, then 101 the following year and 120 (nearly 36% of the year's total intake) the year after that. Most of these elderly people were incurable, with diagnoses of brain damage, cerebral arteriosclerosis, or senility; only about one in five was in the potentially recoverable group of manic–depressives. For Dr Last it had been a matter of humanity to respond to the distress of an old person unable to cope on her own, or to help a family with few members living in cramped quarters and all out at work and unable to supervise an old person with failing memory. He admitted them to hospital without reckoning the consequences.

At first no one noticed what was happening. It presented itself as a surprising lack of nurses in the admission wards (they had gone to do the heavy physical nursing of the old women). The geriatric wards were beginning to overflow with extra beds. Most importantly old people who could not be discharged were staying on the admission wards instead of being transferred as formerly to a geriatric ward. They occupied beds needed for new acute, mostly younger patients.

Early in 1967 a census was taken of all women in-patients. There were 369 women in 11 wards, and 110 beds were for heavy geriatric nursing. All but four of these geriatric patients needed help with washing and dressing, three-quarters of them wet themselves day and night unless attended to, half had to be helped with their food, half could not get in or out of bed or walk unaided – and nearly half had already been more than five years in the hospital. The numbers of elderly women in the different wards are shown in Table 12.1. It can be seen that more than half the 369 women were more than 65 years old. There were a further 32 age 60–64. To lift a heavy-nursing patient takes a minimum of two nurses at once. Collectively these old people were soaking up more and more of the available nurses, including students who had signed on to learn about handling behavioural problems rather than heavy incontinents.

Dr Last's policy could not continue. Admissions had to be restricted. Crisis meetings were held with the medical and nursing staff, general practitioners informed, and Dr Rosemary Rue came from the Regional Board to find a solution. This was to agree to additional facilities and staff, but in a new setting which would offer a much greater variety of types of help and at the same time restrict help to the essential. A new distinct department of mental health of the elderly under a new consultant specialist would work partly at St John's and partly at Tindal Hospital in Aylesbury, close to a centre of geriatric medicine. Very great use would be made of day centres, there and elsewhere, and of home visits, especially by psychiatric nurses who would in some cases teach families how to cope. Admission to hospital would mostly be for limited terms only, to give families a short holiday from caring, or for medical assessment and treatment where this could not be given at home.

TABLE 12.1
Numbers of old women in-patients, 1967

	Type of nursing required	No. of beds on wards	Patient numbers		
			aged 65–74	*aged 75–84*	*aged 85 and over*
Two wards	Light nursing	55	24	17	4
Three wards	Heavy nursing	110	25	48	26
Six wards	Chronic mental	204	33	12	3
Totals		369	82	77	33

TABLE 12.2
Assessments, day-patient attendances and domiciliary visits: psychogeriatric patients 1973 and 1981

	Numbers of cases
1973, all Bucks	
Assessments	
Tindal admissions	235
day attendances	67
domiciliary visits by doctor	13
Day patients	
new referrals, Tindal and St John's	142
total attendances[1]	10 000
Nursing domiciliary visits	3364
1981, Aylesbury area only	
Assessments	
Tindal admissions	225
day attendances	115
domiciliary visits by doctor	563
Day patients	
new	62
support care	310

1. Note that a day patient who attends five days a week attends over 250 times a year.

Dr D. M. D. White was appointed to this new post in April 1970. One ward at St John's became a geriatric day hospital and he was allowed 136 beds otherwise, including 23 for short assessment and 22 for holiday breaks. In 1972 a ward of 22 assessment beds opened at Tindal, and later there was a day hospital there too. He was very vigorous in assessments and visits, as the 1973 figures for the new department show (Table 12.2). The nursing visits however were low, owing to the difficulty in recruiting staff.

At the end of 1973 a second consultant was appointed, and a junior doctor seconded part-time from St John's. By 1981 the county had been split into three and each now had its own consultant and staff and its own patients. The work had increased: the 1981 figures for one area alone, Aylesbury, are shown in Table 12.2. The Tindal unit moved to ward 5 at Stoke Mandeville Hospital in 1986, and obtained some new buildings.

The removal of the elderly from the mental hospital was the second time a category of patients had been split off: previously the mentally handicapped had been withdrawn to special facilities, and it was no longer the practice to admit other children since the development of the special Park Hospital for them in Oxford.

The shrinkage of St John's continued. It was down to about 330 in-patients in 1987, some wards were altogether closed, and Beacon House was no longer for admissions but used as a rehabilitation centre.

Where were the nurses?

The nursing shortage of the early 1950s had been alleviated by the recruitment of 50 students to the new nursing school, and by taking on part-time staff willing to work at least nine hours per week. Another new help was the introduction of staff who knew no nursing, housekeepers and ward orderlies who had domestic duties such as cleaning and serving meals. They were counted as nursing staff and could be used in the general supervision of patients if essential. There were also people called nursing assistants who were shown how to help patients feed and dress.

Student nurses had a definite educational standard from school and worked for three years (with at least six months of this in training school) before taking the examination for registered mental nurse (RMN), after passing which they became staff nurses or higher. A few might also become a state-registered nurse (SRN) by studying general nursing after or before their psychiatric course. But there were also pupil nurses, non-academic, given practical instruction in the wards and after two years becoming state-enrolled nurses (SEN) without passing any examinations.

Working with so many pupils and nursing assistants and students threw a heavy burden on the fully trained staff, who had to supervise, instruct, and at the same time learn new techniques themselves. Nursing was becoming both more medical with the introduction of many new drugs, and more psychologically demanding with the development of ideas of a therapeutic community, of group psychotherapy, of behaviour therapy and the like in which nurses were to take part.

It is important to realise that the so-called nursing staff was in fact a very mixed group of people of varying knowledge and experience, only a minority of whom might be nurses in the full sense. Together they kept the hospital afloat, but only just. Recruitment was never easy, and trained nurses were in very short supply.

In the 1960s things began to go wrong again. The medical staff and several Committee members, making inspection visits at 9 p.m. or later, discovered many wards had no night nurse at all. In some cases the patients were locked in by themselves till morning; in others a patrol passed every one or two hours, to make sure things were alright. This luckily caught the beginnings of a fire on one occasion, but not suicides on two others. In different wards men were found hanging in the toilets when a nurse came on duty in the morning. At a Committee visit in March 1964 three wards of men (108 patients) were on their own at night, and seven wards of women with serious overcrowding had no night staff.

By day, nurses became less visible in the acute wards. In one, with 24 newly admitted women under the eye of a single student nurse, a suicide took place at about 11 a.m. A patient slipped away unnoticed, turned on the taps in the bathroom, and drowned herself.

Where had all the nurses gone? There was a total of 145 staff to look after 420 women, working a three-shift day, 7 a.m.–2 p.m., 1.30 p.m.–9 p.m. and 8.30 p.m.–7.30 a.m. But on any given day about 50 staff were unavailable, because it was their day off, or annual leave, or they were sick (an important variable) or away at a teaching course. Others had to be allotted to special activities, occupational or industrial therapy or day hospital or administration. Allowing for this and night duty subtracted another 25. So only about 70 people were available to the wards, for two shifts. But the heavy-nursing wards each needed four or five nurses per shift, leaving about 20 people for the rest of the hospital, where most of the diagnostic and therapeutic work was taking place. Note we have to say people, not nurses, because of the lack of trained staff. This was something administrators and committees were very prone to overlook.

The nursing staff of the hospital was from 1853 rigorously separated into a male and a female side. It still was so in 1967, with male nurses under a chief male nurse and female nurses under a matron: two independent administrations, two separate duty rotas. However, in 1957 female ward orderlies had been introduced on both sides of the hospital and in the 1960s the matron had recruited one or two male nurses to her staff. The two administrations faced rather different problems. The geriatric excess was primarily female, but recruitment of women staff was more difficult than that of male staff. Over five years the male side improved and the female deteriorated (Table 12.3). In five years matron had increased the number of names on her books, but they were all part-time staff. The number of her students declined, the number of trained staff remained static. She had almost half the number of trained nurses the male side disposed of, to cover 20% more patients.

The HMC proved incapable of facing the nursing crisis, which was complicated by a clash of personality between the matron and the chief male nurse. He had been appointed six years before her, they had different social and educational backgrounds, he was independent and a joker, she orderly and serious: a jealous rivalry had developed. They could not agree on a common plan to improve the nursing situation.

The Regional Board, already intervening to solve the problem of the elderly, cut the Gordian knot. The male and female sides had to be integrated into one nursing force, so that any nurse could be posted anywhere his or her skills were most needed, and only one administration would be necessary. To achieve this the matron was given early retirement, and a couple of years later the chief male nurse resigned. This and the gradual withdrawal of the burden of the elderly worked for the time being. But a contemporary

TABLE 12.3
Nursing staff, 1962 and 1967

	For 350 male patients		For 420 female patients	
	1962	*1967*	*1962*	*1967*
Total (all grades)	73	110	129	145
Full-time staff	72	84	97	99
Full-time trained nurses	34	43	22	23
Students	15	28	45	24

TABLE 12.4
Comparison of numbers of nursing staff at St John's and St Crispin's hospitals, 1967

	St John's (770 beds)	St Crispin's (943 beds)
All full-time staff	184	281
trained full-time staff	69	101
students	53	78
Part-time staff	78	53
Total	262	334

comparison of nursing strengths between St John's and St Crispin's mental hospital at Northampton shows that St John's was still badly off (Table 12.4). It is obvious that St Crispin's, with 20% more patients, had more than 20% more full-time, student, and fully trained staff. But administrators and committees like simpler figures, such as the staff:patient ratio. Dividing the totals pares down the difference between them: St John's, with 770 patients and 262 staff, shows a staff:patient ratio of 1:2.9, St Crispin's a ratio of 1:2.8.

But the Regional Board had one further action to take. The sudden death of the St John's chief administrator, the hospital secretary, and of the matron of Stoke Mandeville Hospital, provided the opportunity. The St John's HMC was abolished and the Royal Bucks–Stoke Mandeville group HMC took over, with their secretary and their new principal nurse in charge of St John's as of the other hospitals of the group. This was 1972, but all would change again in 1974, with a major administrative reorganisation of the NHS. The old chronic problems were to land in new in-trays.

Quality control

One day in the late 1960s a doctor had to interview a woman who had been an in-patient for a long time to tell her that her husband had decided to divorce her because she seemed to be incurable. When she came into the office for the interview he noticed she had two severe black eyes, but she was unwilling to talk about them. Neither the daily nor nightly nursing reports made any mention of them, or of any accident or fight, and there was nothing in the accident-report book. The ward sister looked uncomfortable but was unwilling or unable to explain, and the lack of any mention of the black eyes was itself a misdemeanour, whatever the explanation. The Medical Director took the matter up with vigour. He held private interviews with a number of nurses and with other patients in the ward. It emerged that the night nurse had struck the patient, and indeed was known in some circles as a rough woman. The Director thereupon suspended her from duty, and reported her to the HMC with the suggestion that she was unsuitable to nurse psychiatric patients and should be dismissed.

The Committee were upset in two ways. In the first place the Director was *ultra vires*: he was not in charge of the nurses and had no authority to suspend or dismiss staff. Secondly, a nursing union was already making threatening noises on behalf of the nurse and in that day and age a person's job was almost sacrosanct, and dismissal therefore out of the question. (Before 1959 the Medical Superintendent had the power of dismissal in such cases, and the regulations and laws in force put the safety of patients before the security of jobs.) Being upset they brushed aside the Director's inquiry and resolved to make their own forthwith. But none of the nurses who had spoken to Dr Watt in private were willing to come forward and give evidence in public. The Chairman therefore closed the matter and ordered the night nurse to be reinstated at once. Perhaps fortunately, at this point she decided to resign; the matter was hushed up, the good name of the hospital preserved.

This was not the only case of patient abuse to come to light without achieving the publicity of newspaper report. Mentally ill people may need protection from violence, unwanted sex acts and robbery because they are weakened by their illness so that they cannot protest convincingly, or believe their sufferings are merited. Some have delusions of persecution, others believe they have committed crimes and must be punished. The early history of the care of the insane was so filled with cruelty that the Commissioners in Lunacy and inspectors of the Board of Control were always on the look-out for it and prepared to prosecute any guilty staff member if the local committee did not act. Nurses and social workers and related professions have no agreed ethical code as doctors have, embodied in the Hippocratic Oath and enforced by the General Medical Council. Like children, the mentally handicapped, the elderly and the mad need special care, and since the ending of the special controls and of the inspectorate, we need a rethink about watching out for cruelty in all institutions, homes, hostels and day centres as well as hospitals, and a proper policy of what to do when it is discovered.

The work in 1974

There is a zone in history where the past merges with the present, where the day before yesterday is still a part of contemporary confusion yet already a part of the record. The year 1974 is a useful boundary in British psychiatric history because the NHS administrative reorganisation then effectively dethroned the asylum, removed it from its central position in the mental health services, and opened the way to its demise.

Before that year the hospital was run by a voluntary committee with the consultants, the principal nursing officers, and the hospital administrators taking many of the decisions, subject to the financial control and approval of the Regional Board. After that year the voluntary committee no longer existed, decision-making was largely taken from the hospital staff and to some extent also from the Regional Board, and a new stratum of professional managers created close to the hospital but outside it: the District Health

Authority, as it became established and confirmed in 1982. These managers were not bound by the horizon of the psychiatric hospital, but saw and co-ordinated all the mental-health provisions, clinics, day centres, hostels, special facilities for children, for the old, for drug addicts and the antisocial and so on. The hospital became only one facility among many. So 1974 is a point from which to look back to the changes since 1961, and forward to closure in 1991.

Since 1961 the Bucks population had expanded in 13 years by nearly 50%, and the annual intake of in-patients risen by 30%, to 858 at St John's, and 137 in the 24-bed ward for psychiatry at Wycombe General Hospital in 1974. New out-patients had risen from 760 to nearly 1200, proportionate to the population increase. The day-patient service, non-existent in 1961, saw 91 new cases attending St John's itself in 1974, plus 135 at Byron House; 36 attended the ward at Wycombe, and 145 at Harlow House; a separate day hospital in Wycombe opened the previous year. The four child guidance clinics saw 426 new cases between them, as against 119 in 1961. These figures do not include the work of the department of mental health of the elderly, nor of course many other activities such as pastoral and domiciliary visits.

These increases were made possible by increases in the medical staff. The consultants had gone up from five to 13 (three wholly for child work, plus two for the elderly and one for mental handicap). There were six new junior doctors, one at registrar level, and five senior house officers, so that child psychiatry and psychogeriatrics could have a registrar each and the Wycombe ward have two house officers. In addition, four general practitioners (GPs) acted as clinical assistants, giving four half-days each. The area had three full-time psychologists and seven social workers provided by the Bucks Social Services Department. In 1969 the staff had been divided into three equal teams, each with a similar set of wards in the hospital and serving a defined third of the county, north, central or south, with equal populations. This was a further step in the decentralisation of services. Each team worked independently, in its own way. Of course doctors differed in the patients they selected for admission, in the length of time they kept them in hospital, and in the extent to which they used the different facilities, and comparison between the teams brought this out for discussion. But analysis of how the team system was working showed that in addition, the three geographical divisions of equal population produced different numbers of patients for the psychiatrist. Why this was so was not investigated: it could have been because GPs in the three areas differed in their practice of referring cases to psychiatrists; or perhaps the populations differed in their age structure or social make-up. But it meant a certain flexibility was needed in sharing out available resources.

Laboratory research was strengthened by the appointment of Dr Peter Bond as a biochemist and of Dr R. Cundall as a clinical psychiatrist with an interest in biochemical work, and investigations of blood enzymes in psychosis resulted.

The emphasis on medical teaching led to the appointment of one of the consultants (in rotation) as clinical tutor, with the equivalent of one day per week to organise courses and tailor the individual junior doctor's opportunities for experience to his or her particular requirements. There was secondment to the adolescent unit at Oxford as well as work in child guidance, mental handicap, or the care of the elderly. GPs in three-year training schemes were offered three or six months' psychiatric experience. Oxford offered day-release lecture courses and supervised the training of senior registrars by a rotation. For a number of years the hospital accepted part-time trainees under the Oxford Region's scheme to bring married women back into medicine when their children were beginning to grow up. A small stream of women doctors began to learn psychiatry, some of them successfully passing the specialist examinations and eventually becoming consultants; one became Director of Prison Medical Services. The old connection with Maudsley post-graduates came to an end, but over the years a selection of overseas doctors came and stayed to work for a time, from Czechoslovakia, Egypt, Spain, Iraq, Argentina, Mauritius, Burma, Pakistan and of course Australia.

Into the '80s

The northern area of the county included the rapidly growing city of Milton Keynes which was soon to get its own hospital beds and day centres. The central area included Manor House Hospital in Aylesbury, opened 1926, for the mentally handicapped and long a poor relation. Although under the same HMC as St John's (but supervised from Borocourt Hospital near Reading) neither Dr Last nor Dr Watt had had any responsibility for it. With the 1974 reorganisation, however, it was brought into the Aylesbury Vale family, and Dr Watt exerted himself to see it get its own consultant in charge who would provide a service to the whole district and not simply care for in-patients. It proved very difficult to find the right person, but after a long time the post was filled. Within St John's itself the years after 1974 showed the inception of a mother-and-baby unit, of a lithium clinic, and of a pre-senile dementia unit. A male nurse started a new wave of rehabilitation, tackling the more difficult patients who had previously responded poorly. An interesting innovation was that the money to pay for this was raised by appealing to local societies for charitable gifts. Beacon House, which had ceased to be needed for new admissions, became, as a result of this initiative, the base for a new rehabilitation team of doctors, psychologist, nurses, occupational therapist and social worker.

The old town of Buckingham became the seat of an interesting five-year experiment in 1984 with the encouragement of Dr Watt and Professor Shepherd. Dr Ian Falloon from the Maudsley Hospital, who had previously carried out research on schizophrenia at St John's, set out to manage all the psychiatric problems of the area by domiciliary and day-centre methods, with himself the only doctor (at first) and his colleagues limited to nurses. Progress was monitored, and among other aims it was hoped to show how far psychiatric illness could be managed with a minimum of medical input and without the use of in-patient beds.

When St John's closes the patients of the central (Aylesbury Vale) area will have a new 50-bed hospital and a day centre on the old Tindal Hospital site, and accommodation for long-stay patients across the road at the Manor House site. It remains to be seen whether this will prove adequate, how the staff will be trained in the new setting, and perhaps most important of all whether recruitment will suffice. The future holds not only doubts about the adequacy of funds for mental health services, but about enough educated people coming forward from a declining population to fill the different professional roles. The progress of medicine is such that we can achieve all sorts of miracles, but the cost of the equipment and staff is becoming so great that we may have to select very severely the miracles we most want. Research to discover the cheapest and simplest way of effective treatment becomes increasingly needed.

Psychiatric help of some kind is being offered to more than one person in every 500 of the population every year, and the demands made of the mental health services have widened to include marriage counselling, forensic advice in court cases and all kinds of problems from the cradle to the grave. The asylum of 1853, and the mental hospital of 1919, have become quite irrelevant. The danger is that in widening the work of the mental health services we forget the most serious sufferers for whom the services originally began: the mad, the psychotic, the chronically disabled.

Notes

After 1974 social workers were no longer a part of the hospital staff, but came from the Social Services Department of the Bucks County Council, as its director thought fit. There was at first a difficult, uncomprehending relationship between the medical and the social services, which improved with a change of director.

13 Looking back

In earlier centuries mental troubles, it was thought, had been produced by the Devil, or the baneful influence of the stars, or the actions of witches. If there was to be treatment it would come from spiritual healers and the religious, or from astrologers who could cast horoscopes and predict the future, or from witch hunters. But in the 18th century in Britain beliefs in witches and the Devil declined while belief in medicines, blood-letting, and other bodily actions mounted. These treatments were not the prerogatives of medical doctors, but the practice of a whole range of self-made specialists, who sometimes advertised in the newspapers.

Among all the people with mental troubles of one kind or another there were some, but only some, who were impossible to live with. Their disordered minds led to disordered behaviour which threatened the life of the home and the family – by attacks on family members or destruction of family property. People were prevented from a night's sleep or from going to work, or found their rooms fouled or windows smashed, or their neighbours the subject of provocative abuse or worse. The mad men or women who did these things had to be restrained. They were tied up, locked in, sometimes provided with guards. If the family could afford it they were sent away to one of the private madhouses run as businesses by enterprising people. These private institutions were of all kinds, mostly small but a few large, some cheap and some very expensive, mostly taking the well-to-do but a few also taking a proportion of paupers, their fees being paid by their parishes. Madness was no respecter of social class: the nobility and gentry were quite as likely to produce a madman as were the labourers and unskilled factory workers, but at least they had the money to cope with it.

Some of these private houses were good, some were dreadful. Over the century 1744–1845 Parliament endeavoured to control them by licensing, inspections, and demanding the keeping of good records. People were encouraged to club together in charitable subscription to establish public institutions which could take all social classes and be run in an open, humane way. Thus the Gloucester County Asylum (opened 1823) and the

Northamptonshire Asylum (opened 1838) took both fee-paying private patients and the poor supported by their parishes. It was only in the 1860s and 1870s, when the asylums had grown enormous, that at Gloucester the private patients were separated at Barnwood House, while at Northampton they remained on the original site as St Andrew's, and the poor were transferred to a new public asylum to be ultimately St Crispin's. The Bucks County Pauper Lunatic Asylum, built when the Act of 1845 made it compulsory to do so, although intended for the poor by priority, also up to 1948 took a few private patients, at the cheaper end of the market. The paying patient could hope for better food, could wear his own clothes, might get a little more of the usually scanty nursing attention, and at least in the more expensive places would not have to mix with the poor and social inferiors, at a time when such class divisions were more important than they are today.

Repeatedly, inspection of the mad in private institutions and in public workhouses revealed that they got very poor medical attention. Doctors were only casually and infrequently called to see them, although severe mental illness gave rise to fractures, cuts, ulcerations and other injuries, some self-inflicted, others acquired in fights or from restraint by chains. The mad were often self-neglectful and malnourished. When brought together in the same building they became good soil for the spread of dysentery, tuberculosis, and infectious fevers. Although mentally ill to start with, they produced much ordinary medical and surgical illness which was frequently neglected. The Act of 1845 specified that any institution of 100 or more inmates must have a doctor on the regular staff.

At first the doctor was not necessarily the director of the asylum. Private places were quite often run by non-doctors. For the first 40 years of its existence the famous Retreat at York had a layman as chief, but then went over to a medical superintendent. The asylums at Bodmin and Bedford tried a lay governor, and so did Hanwell in Middlesex for a time after Dr Conolly resigned. Lay chiefs were not found to be satisfactory in practice, and there was an obvious saving in money in making a resident doctor responsible for everything. Lord Shaftesbury became converted to the idea. The non-restraint movement, which got rid of the handcuffs and chains so long and so widely used in controlling the mad, was the work of doctors such as Gaskell, Charlesworth, Gardiner Hill and Conolly, followed by others such as Mr Millar at Stone. The doctor was made legally responsible for the patients, and the chief employee under the magistrates' committee which financed and ran the place. He was a social inferior to the country gentlemen.

It was only after the Medical Reform Act 1858, which created a medical register on which only those of approved training who had passed professional examinations could be inscribed, that the medical profession generally began to rise in public esteem. Before that anyone could claim to be a doctor and practise, even quite irresponsibly, and it was hard for the public to tell the good and the bad apart. Among doctors, however, the asylum or mental hospital doctor, and even the psychiatrist of today, remained for a very long time at the social bottom of the medical profession. The poor status of Mr Humphry and Dr Kerr is shown by the way they were denied medical assistance and overloaded with work in overcrowded buildings in spite of recurrent pressure from the Commissioners in Lunacy on the Committee of magistrates to do something about it. The doctors had no power to refuse anyone the magistrates chose to send in. There is no sign of them building up their professional stake, boosting the importance of medical psychiatry, gaining more power in their world. Between 1860 and 1930, say, British asylums remained backwaters. They were closely controlled by laymen; they were a part of local government, not a state service, till 1948.

There are historians who discern a mental hospital movement of ambitious medical men carving out a new specialty for themselves and claiming mental trouble as an illness so they could make the mad their exclusive property. There is very little sign of this in British history, and none in Bucks. There are Marxist sociologists convinced that asylums were created to threaten the common people and keep them quietly working in the factories of the capitalist establishment; convinced too that mental disturbance was only a label attached to the social deviant, the rebel, to neutralise him and maintain the status quo. Again, the facts of English history do not support these beliefs. Perhaps in other countries with different forms of government, different political and religious beliefs, and different social cultures, the history of the mad and of asylums may be different. Madness is international, but what is done about it is a practical expression of local belief. Whatever may have been in France and Germany, in England the public asylum grew out of a need of families to be relieved of the burden of severely disturbed relatives, and a wish to offer to the poor what the rich were already buying for themselves. It grew out of the same compassion which sought to free slaves, limit the working of children in factories, help orphans and fallen women: the Victorian Christian charitable drive.

Lord Shaftesbury was an evangelical Christian who fought for all these causes and ruled the Lunacy Commission for 40 years. His influence no doubt made the Commissioners inquire frequently for the proportion of patients attending the (Anglican) church services regularly, and urge an increase in their numbers; when the asylum began to expand they were quick to urge the magistrates to build a new and much bigger chapel. Great value was put upon religion as a form of treatment, a kind of psychotherapy. The chaplain at Bucks was the best-paid asylum officer after the superintendent and the steward, and got the pay later thought appropriate for an assistant medical officer. He had much more to do than hold two services a week – he had to visit all wards and all patients regularly. Some people held to the idea that mental illness was due to intemperance and vicious habits, and later that the life of pauperism itself was somehow morally wrong.

The Bucks asylum of 1853 was a sunny, airy building with a southerly view to the Chiltern Hills and modern (gas) lighting, central heating, baths and wash-basins with hot and cold running water, and toilets. It was furnished to a high standard, provided with good food, and run openly without restraints. Patients were encouraged to go out and mix in society. Mr Millar tried to lead his doubting Committee in the path of humanity and freedom, but he was let down by his chief male nurse and the magistrates turned against him. After his fall, the high standards of domestic care began to slip, and the cost of everything to become a major concern.

But there was already a change in public attitude. Bringing the mad together in asylums after 1845 made them altogether more visible, as they went for country walks in large groups with their nurses, or wandered in the fenced gardens of their enormous eye-catching institutions. There seemed to be so many of them, far more than people had thought, the numbers ever rising, and some of them chronically and horribly disabled. The early asylums had been on a small domestic scale and the Lunacy Commission urged keeping them like that. They advised building new small asylums to house the growing numbers. But it was cheaper to go on enlarging existing buildings, even up to ten times, turning them into separate walled villages, and that is what happened.

Fear and horror were replacing compassion. The image of the lunatic as a dangerous murderer grew. People were frightened by the possibility that a normal person could be wrongly imprisoned with the lunatics. Public opposition grew to letting patients out and about in the community, and leave was curtailed. Patients were forced to retreat behind the walls of their asylums, to become isolated from the community around them, as to a lesser extent did those who looked after them. Meanwhile the doctors, faced with so many new patients and the evils of overcrowding and understaffing, emphasised every year the growing burden of incurable cases, no doubt to encourage their committees to provide more facilities. They glossed over the fact that 30% or more of those admitted to the asylum went home again quite soon, many within six months.

The Lunacy (Consolidation) Act 1890 expressed the dominant fear and pessimism; make sure the mad are really mad, and then shut them out of society; provide careful legal machinery to make admission to asylum safe and sure and don't worry after that – few of them can be trusted to be let out again. At the same time control passed from the magistrates, the well-to-do country gentlemen, to the democratically elected county councillors, some of them successful tradesmen, some of them Nonconformists by religion, some of them with a view of paupers as lazy good-for-nothings, a town rather than a country view. The first thing the new rulers did, not only in Bucks, was to cancel the patients' beer ration and substitute water. The next was to make financial savings by cutting down on their food. If they were paupers, anything more than the bare essentials for survival was unnecessary, was spoiling them. When it came to World War I the finance committees cut the food some more in the face of rising prices. Bucks seems to have been one of the most severe in this, and many patients died as a result; but concern was very muted, and the deaths hushed up.

The county councillors could be proud of a big new building, of a modern electric kitchen with gleaming meters and control knobs, of an experimental farm on the hospital's land, but as for the inmates, that was the doctors' affair – the rubbish of society had to go somewhere. The asylums had started as places where it was hoped to cure people, but an increasing number of incurables had come to light and had to be kept alive. The institution which had prided itself on being well above a workhouse, with a different philosophy behind it, had sunk to workhouse level. The idea of therapy had been largely forgotten; perhaps the few doctors had no time to think about this, or to explain to laymen what might be done, if indeed they were not ignorant themselves. The advances in psychiatry came from abroad, principally from German-speaking countries where study of and teaching about mental illness was a university subject, while British doctors had little teaching and less thinking to sustain them. But why did they fail to convince the councillors that attempts to stop tuberculosis could be very successful, that they could save lives instead of destroying them, at a small cost to the county rates?

The accumulation of incurables had several causes, and could have been better understood if it had been investigated. Part of the explanation was demographic. The population of England was expanding, living longer, and more babies, especially the mentally handicapped, were surviving into childhood and adult life thanks to bacteriology and public health measures. Perhaps those already staying in the asylum lived there longer than of yore, instead of dying off. Schizophrenia as a disease may have fluctuated in incidence, though this does not seem to be the case in Bucks. It was certainly a fact that people who did not need to be in the asylum lingered there, because amid the crowd no one noticed they had recovered, or there was no incentive to discharge them, but rather a tendency to play safe and hang on to them in case they broke down again.

World War I, the Great War, which put millions of men into uniform, produced a great crop of mental illnesses. Soldiers who became psychotic were transferred to asylums as private (service) patients paid for by the Government. In popular view at least this madness was caused by the hellish conditions of the Flanders front-line, and was a matter of compassion. Neurotic illnesses of various kinds burgeoned also, without physical causes but perhaps from some kind of emotional block. There was a new medical interest in such matters. The work of Freud in Vienna and of Jung in Zurich began to filter through, to the public as well as the doctors. There were also successful physical treatments: malarial fever therapy for general paralysis of the insane in 1917, and barbiturate drugs for epilepsy in 1912, two conditions responsible between them for a good many asylum in-patients (and long departed from the psychiatric hospital of today). The result was a new public attitude. Mental illness might have emotional roots rather than arising from poverty, and it was not incurable in essence but there was hope of recovery, in the future if not now.

The new attitude was expressed by the Royal Commission of 1926 and confirmed in the Mental Treatment Act 1930. Treatment of all the mentally ill, not just the certifiable, must be the aim, and they must no longer be segregated. Asylums must open up and offer treatment to all who wanted it, and other hospitals too, as well as out-patient clinics, must help the mentally afflicted. Doors were to be unlocked, patients come and go without legal formality, and the old image of the prison camp filled with long-stay inmates mopping and mowing under the gaze of men in paramilitary uniform (or even white coats) was to be expunged forever from the mental health services.

The change in reality was slow, and the Bucks County Mental Hospital under Skottowe in the 1930s and '40s was a leader in it. But it was only in the '50s, with the better finance and technical understanding brought by the NHS, that the Act of 1930 came to fruition. The change depended in part on technical developments in everyday life, particularly the telephone and the motorcar, which altered the way in which a medical service operated; the computer and the fax machine will alter it again, with new possibilities. But it also depended on the emergence of new professions, such as social workers, to take part in an increasing complexity of diagnostic and therapeutic management. The 1959 Act and the 1983 Act carried things further in the same direction; magistrates ceased to have any role, admission and discharge after very few weeks without more formality than in a general hospital became the rule. Alternatives to hospital admission developed. Freedom and respect for civil rights, psychological as well as physical treatment, became the new order. University teaching and research and training courses across the country improved the quality of what was done. But the public image of the asylum lingered on. In the '60s patients admitted to the new acute ward, Beacon House, which stood in the grounds of St John's about 50 yards across the grass from the old building, strongly maintained they were in a different hospital and spoke with horror and mistrust of what they imagined (quite wrongly) went on in the main building. University teachers in the arts, writers and journalists and television producers, felt fully qualified to inform the world that psychiatry had not advanced since 1880, contained no body of knowledge and was obviously on the wrong track. Antipsychiatry blossomed.

No doubt some of its emotional roots are those which make people anti-science and anti-doctor in general: fear of what man will do to man in the torture chamber, of what we may do to one another with radioactivity and chemical pollution, of the power of the medico to dehumanise one and see one as a flawed machine. There are also professional roots, as the psychologists, social workers, graduate nurses and others assert their independence from the medical profession and promote their own special contributions to mental health problems.

Intellectually, there is a failure to understand the nature of medical science in two aspects. One is that it proceeds not from theory, from intellectual penetration or intuition, but from human experience. The successful treatment with electroconvulsive shock arises from the observation that some asylum patients got better after suffering spontaneously an epileptic fit: hence epileptic fits might make some others better. Who could have thought this would be so? The fact that over 50 years later we do not know why it is so detracts in no way from the treatment; medicine is full of such empirical but valuable knowledge. We do not know why aspirin works, but we are quite prepared to swallow it. Science proceeds from ever-widening experience, helped by new instruments and chance encounters. This is the second overlooked aspect. Science proceeds – it is not a static subject. Mankind has accumulated a great deal of psychiatric information since 1880, and particularly since 1950, and this will go on and on if social conditions allow. The pundits who tell us nothing has changed simply do not understand how it does change; they are looking in the stars for a new philosophy instead of at wretched humans in a hospital ward.

Since 1850 we have advanced in several distinct ways. Detailed observations of behaviour in hospital and clinic have allowed division of the mentally ill into groups with different prognoses, whose life will unfold differently, and in some cases with the ability to get better with special treatment. In some of these it has been possible to link their mental illness to some physical condition, an abnormality in endocrine or vitamin function, a form of cancer, an enzyme deficiency, a blood vascular disturbance. Correction of the physical may then relieve the mental. In a series of accidents drugs have been discovered with powerful effects on limited aspects of mental symptoms and functions.

We have also advanced in understanding the promotion and extinction of learning, and in making use of man's interaction with man in therapy. Individual psychotherapy apart, we are much more aware of the way societies live and put pressures on individuals, sometimes with bad effects. But we are still fumbling over the way to organise and administer a mental health service that is effective, adequate, economic and humane. Our history shows that those who control the money supply effectively decide what is done, yet often lack the detailed or technical knowledge to decide correctly to achieve desired ends. One problem of the 1990s is how to recruit, train and combine the various professionals and their necessary technical equipment into a harmonious effective team which can support and cure the mentally ill even to the extent now possible, let alone taking advantage of future scientific discoveries.

The mid-Victorian asylum was based on a large family, with the superintendent as father, but quickly outgrew the capacity to function. The current model is the hotel chain or high-street supermarket, where the ill person is a customer not a relation. We are still discovering the drawbacks of this pattern, but one of them appears to be that it works badly with those who have lost their normal understanding and power of self-determination. The seriously depressed person may commit suicide unless prevented; the schizophrenic will let everything slide in indifference or indecision, or simply from lack of energy, and may need maternal or paternal care to survive. There is still a need for a social psychology of health administration to teach us how to do better.

Notes

Ackerknecht (1959) gives a brief outline of 19th-century and early 20th-century developments in French and German psychiatry. Levitt (1976) describes the changes made to the NHS in 1976. Allderidge (1979, 1985) provides good further reading.

ACKERKNECHT, E. H. (1959) *Short History of Psychiatry* (trans. S. Wolff). New York: Hefner.
ALLDERIDGE, P. (1979) Hospitals, madhouses and asylums: cycles in the care of the insane. *British Journal of Psychiatry*, **134**, 321–334.
—— (1985) Bedlam: fact or fantasy. In *The Anatomy of Madness*, vol. 2 (eds W. F. Bynum, R. Porter & M. Shepherd). London: Tavistock.
LEVITT, R. (1976) *The Reorganised National Health Service*. London: Croom Helm.

V. Appendix

The future

The rational basis for the closure of St John's Hospital, the old Pauper County Lunatic Asylum, in 1991, includes the following four points.

(a) The great increase in the population of the county has led to a split into three roughly equal areas with separate health service districts. Aylesbury Vale, including the towns of Aylesbury and Buckingham and the country around, is one of them.

(b) Effective treatments have come into being and can be offered to a much wider group of ill people than before. The old asylum catered only for a limited number, the severely disabled, the epileptic, the mentally handicapped, and the elderly. They are often managed now in other units, or in some cases have ceased to exist (cases of GPI, for instance).

(c) Treatment requires the work of many different professions, not just doctors and attendants and nurses.

(d) Modern communications mean many patients can come daily for treatment but continue to live at home, which is often preferable.

Dr Julian Candy (Chairman of the Division of Psychiatry, 1985–89) has contributed the following account.

Mental health services for Aylesbury Vale in 1991 and beyond

Over the past few years we have been developing a comprehensive and up-to-date mental health service for Aylesbury Vale. For us, the closure of St John's is not an aim but a consequence of plans to establish locally based psychiatric services throughout Buckinghamshire.

Since 1974 health care in Buckinghamshire has been provided by three district health authorities: Milton Keynes in the north, Aylesbury Vale in the centre, and Wycombe in the south of the county. Each authority is charged with providing all aspects of specialist health care for its resident population. St John's Hospital, however, was established as the county asylum to receive patients from the whole of Buckinghamshire, from places as far apart as Olney in the north and Marlow 70 miles away in the south. Modern methods of treating mental illness mean that most of those patients who need hospital care stay for no more than a few weeks. Thus for patients (and relatives) to travel so far is not only inconvenient but hampers proper care and rehabilitation. Moreover, Buckinghamshire's population, especially in Milton Keynes and Wycombe, those parts most distant from St John's, is one of the fastest growing in the country. For these reasons, among others, Oxford Regional Health Authority resolved in 1983 to fund and support the development of local and comprehensive mental health services in each of the three Buckinghamshire health districts. Once these developments are in place, St John's Hospital, no longer suitable for modern care in site, size or design, will have served its turn, and can close.

What facilities will then be available for the specialist mental health care of the people of Aylesbury Vale, who number about 155 000? We will continue to provide separate services for people under 65 when they first need care, and for those falling ill over the age of 65. Further, the towns of Buckingham and Winslow will have their own facilities. At Tindal Hospital in Aylesbury town (named after the Clerk of the Peace who was secretary to the magistrates who planned and ran St John's in its early days) will stand a newly built 50-bed unit for people under 65 who need hospital care for a few weeks or months. Two beds for mothers with their babies and two secure rooms for the short-term care of severely disturbed patients will be provided on these wards. A resource centre, providing day-time treatment for up to 30 people well enough to live at home, will occupy part of the same site. Across the road at Manor House Hospital will be a ward for 12 patients with pre-senile dementia, together with about 25 beds for patients from the whole of Buckinghamshire who have been in St John's for many years and are not well enough to leave hospital.

Some mental illness facilities will remain on the St John's Hospital site, though most of it will be sold. Beacon House will become home for a further 60 or so long-stay patients. Next to Beacon House our industrial therapy unit will be rebuilt.

At present people partly handicapped or recovering from serious mental illness are accommodated in 13 'group homes' offering about 50 places in all. These have no living-in staff, though all residents receive regular help and supervision from social workers, community psychiatric nurses, and doctors. Many of these homes are managed by voluntary organisations. Likewise, social services and voluntary bodies provide about 35 places within Aylesbury Vale in partly or fully staffed hostels for people with mental illness, and we have access to further places outside the district. Fortunately, in the field of mental health Buckinghamshire has a tradition of fruitful partnership between health and social services and the voluntary sector.

Since 1984 Buckingham and Winslow, towns in the north of the district with a population of about 33 000, have been served by a community mental health team. This team numbers about 14 in all, made up of a psychiatrist, nurse therapists, community psychiatric nurses, a psychologist, an occupational therapist and a social worker. They work very closely with general practitioners (GPs), and aim to care for even acutely ill patients in their own homes or other domestic settings, thus whenever possible avoiding admission to hospital. This innovative pattern of care is being evaluated by the Department of Health, and has developed a reputation in the UK and abroad.

More recently three community mental health teams have been set up to serve Aylesbury itself and the surrounding villages. These provide specialist psychiatric care for people under 65 who are on the lists of particular GPs. (For the small but important group of mentally ill people not registered with a GP, and perhaps without a settled way of life, allocation to a team is related to their address at first contact.) Again, each team comprises doctors, community psychiatric nurses, psychologists, occupational therapists, social workers, and rehabilitation officers. All members visit patients in their own homes when appropriate, and the doctors see out-patient referrals either in the hospital setting or in GP surgeries. However, there is less emphasis than in Buckingham and Winslow on domiciliary care, and the full range of in-patient, day patient, out-patient and home-based services is employed.

A small specialist team comprising part-time medical, nursing and psychology staff will form part of a wider multi-agency service to people with significant alcohol and drug-related problems.

A separate service (the Department of Mental Health of the Elderly) provides for the needs of those over 65 at first referral. A 24-bed short-stay ward on the Stoke Mandeville Hospital site, with an adjacent 40-place day hospital, has recently been opened. Next to Beacon House on the edge of the old St John's Hospital site, a 35-place privately managed but partly NHS-funded home for elderly people with longer-term mental illness is being built. The number of private residential and nursing homes offering care for elderly people with mental illness has been increasing in recent years, and further co-operative ventures may be undertaken.

Similar developments are under way in Milton Keynes and Wycombe health districts. When all these projects are completed, in each district almost all aspects of psychiatric care will be available locally. A particular exception is care for patients requiring secure accommodation short of a special hospital such as Broadmoor. For Buckinghamshire such patients go to Marlborough House, the 10-bed regional secure unit in Milton Keynes.

Index